MW01591244

Good Word. Good Food. Good Health:

A Clear and Simple Food and Nutrition Handbook

William L. Toples

Cover design by Ms. Kendra Wells, Ardnek 3d

Editing services by CreateSpace

All scripture quotations are taken from the Holy Bible utilizing the New International Version (NIV), Zondervan Bible Publishers, Grand Rapids, MI

Publisher: William L. Toples

Author's web address: www.goodwordfoodhealth.com
Author's e-mail address: wtoples@goodwordfoodhealth.com

ISBN 10: 1518607314
ISBN 13: 9781518607318

Library of Congress Control Number: 2015917056
CreateSpace Independent Publishing Platform
North Charleston, South Carolina

ACKNOWLEDGMENTS

This book is dedicated to eternal God Jehovah, and to my Lord and Savior, Jesus, who provided the divine purpose and inspiration for this work!

The book is also dedicated to the love of my life, my wife of thirty-eight years, Vera Jane, who, through her courage and strength in fighting the tremendous challenges of breast cancer, provided the inspiration to research critically important and understandable information for those seeking to have greater health through nutrition. Her journey gave this work wings!

I extend my love and a very special acknowledgment to my beautiful daughter, Ashleigh Kristina, a true joy and inspiration in my life, whose prayers helped me to complete this assignment and who also provided the title for this work and requested specific research on certain foods; thank you!

I would also like to say thank you and express my love to my mother, Anna Laura, for all of her prayers and sacrifices and for safely protecting and guiding me in my earlier years, and I express that same love to my sisters and my brother: Victoria, a mentor and recent author who offered great ideas and guided me through the publishing process; Portia, an accomplished author who closely reviewed the original manuscript and provided outstanding support; Nedenia, the youngest sister, who often asked if the book was finished and is a great blessing to our family; and my wonderful brother, Johnny, who lives in eternal peace!

I would be remiss not to give a loving shout-out to my nieces, nephews, great-nieces, great-nephews, cousins, in-laws, friends, church family, and extended family members who I pray are inspired by this work and now recognize that God can use each of us for his divine will and purpose! A warm remembrance will always be in my heart for those friends and family members who have gone on to their reward, many of whose shoulders I stand on today.

I would like to thank and acknowledge Blue Cross Blue Shield of Michigan and my brothers at 100 Black Men of Greater Detroit, who together are doing great work in supporting the health of African American men and their families throughout metropolitan Detroit!

A special thank-you to Ms. Kendra Wells, Ardnek 3d, for her excellent work in creating the book-cover designs.

Thank you also to CreateSpace for their editing and design services.

I pray that God continues to bless each of you and your families and that all of your needs are met according to his perfect will, and I express my profound gratitude for having shared this journey with you!

CONTENTS

FOREWORD

I've spent a career dedicated to health and wellness. In urban communities, there are significant challenges with people having a clear understanding of how nutritional choices impact health and wellness. In the book *Good Word. Good Food. Good Health: A Clear and Simple Food and Nutrition Handbook*, Mr. William L. Toples does an outstanding job in sharing the value of good eating habits and the positive impact it can have on the quality of your life. In my medical practice, I see the positive effects of better food choices. The book validates this reality.

Many people want to make good nutrition choices; however, they may lack the necessary knowledge and insight relating to why it's important to be committed to good eating habits. As I read the book, it was clear that Mr. Toples had been thorough in his considerable research related to healthy eating habits. His knowledge of this important topic was evident and profound. What I really found to be amazing is that the approach suggested by Mr. Toples is sustainable, in that by making a few changes in food choices, you can enhance your health and the health of your family. The book is written in a way that everyday people can read and understand the importance of healthy food choices. While the book is an important resource for the health-care profession, it is also essential for the community at large.

Over the years in working with Mr. Toples through our affiliation with the 100 Black Men of Greater Detroit (the 100), an organization committed to enhancing the quality of life of the African American community, Mr. Toples was highly engaged in leading the health and wellness agenda. He worked tirelessly in developing and implementing programs to raise public awareness of the importance of developing a healthy lifestyle and eating habits.

As we worked together in the 100, it was clear to me that Mr. Toples was a leader, champion, and advocate for enhancing awareness and gaining commitment, support, and sponsorship for programs that promoted health and wellness, with a particular focus in the African American community. This effort truly resonated with me, as I also share a passion for health and wellness in the urban community. I believe this book brings an important and critical message regarding the role of nutrition in relationship to sustaining health and reducing chronic health conditions.

As a result of reading the book, here are just a few nuggets of truth that readers can expect to learn. First, the value of whole food such as fresh fruits, vegetables, beans, grains, and other whole foods and their companion phytonutrients, vitamins, and minerals is richly described; their monumental importance in our daily eating habits and overall health and wellness is a truth that clearly emerges in the book. Second, food choices that restrict saturated fats, limit processed food with high levels of added salt and sugar, and avoid trans fats and questionable food additives are critical decisions for sustaining health. Third, you are accountable for your food choices—you can make better choices by increasing your knowledge with the important information contained in the book. Fourth, food is for strengthening our bodies to complete assignments given to us in accordance with our calling and purpose. In addition, the importance of proper water intake is an added insight shared in the book; proper hydration is critical in reducing many common health issues.

A favorite chapter in the book is "If Body Parts Could Talk." This chapter is presented in an easy-to-understand manner in which readers can appreciate the essential role of human organs and the proper nutrition and care required for these important body components. These are just a few insights that make this book required reading. I urge you to read the entire book to gain valuable insight concerning better food choices for increased health and wellness.

In closing, I am honored to write the foreword and want to congratulate Mr. Toples for his outstanding work and for bringing this important book to the community. Let me suggest that health and nutrition is a process. It takes time, effort, knowledge, and energy. For this reason, I am aligned with and committed to the efforts of Mr. Toples; he has provided support for getting to a life of increased health, which can ultimately bring about more meaningful outcomes in the communities in which we serve. As a practicing physician and health-care professional, I recognize that health and wellness enhances your quality of life. As such, you can gain vital insight through reading this important book, *Good Word. Good Food. Good Health: A Clear and Simple Food and Nutrition Handbook.* It can get you on the path to better knowledge, better eating, and better health.

Herbert C. Smitherman Jr., MD, MPH, FACP
Interim Vice Dean, Diversity and Inclusion
Assistant Dean, Community and Urban Health
Associate Professor, Department of Medicine
and Karmanos Cancer Institute
Wayne State University School of Medicine/Detroit Medical Center
President and CEO, Health Centers Detroit Foundation, Inc.

INTRODUCTION

Like a lot of new authors, I didn't start out to write a book—particularly one about such a very broad and engulfing topic as food and nutrition. However, the events that led up to this endeavor were so sobering and inspiring that they surpassed the notion of "if" and transcended into a question and emotion of "how."

I refer to this endeavor as "clear and simple" not to suggest this information lacks true value or a depth of sincerity, but to reinforce the idea that important information, such as food and nutrition, is oftentimes at the bottom of the book pile because of the overly scientific and cumbersome way in which it is presented. After three or four pages of scientific mumbo jumbo associated with amino-acid strands, it's no wonder why one of the most important books remains at the bottom of the pile. It's also no wonder when the book contains 350 pages of uninspiring, ant-size type and graphs.

With the help of the Creator, I will attempt to impart knowledge in a very clear, simple, and concise manner, using as few scientific explanations and in as few pages as humanly possible, concerning the nutrition of everyday and common foods that you likely consume regularly. I will be very transparent in stating that I am not a licensed nutritionist or dietician, and the following pages are in no way intended as an all-encompassing fact book and final record about every scientific aspect of food and nutrition; I am not that full of my talents and abilities, nor is that the goal of this book. Rather, I am very comfortable in stating that this is a work that comes from widely available information, assembled for people looking for vital yet basic food and nutrition information, presented in an understandable and unintimidating way. The richest part of this book is centered on and describes plant-based "whole" food.

Moving on, I would like to share a brief story about an important and life-changing event concerning my wife, Vera—a story that too many women have experienced. Vera was diagnosed with breast cancer in the earlier part of 2006. My wife informed me of this shortly after she learned of the issue, and soon after that, she informed our daughter, Ashleigh Kristina. Needless to say, we were all very surprised by this revelation and wondered how we would proceed with tackling such a major health challenge. Family, friends, church members, neighbors, and coworkers were informed shortly thereafter, which created a very strong support network that we shall never forget and that has lasted through this very writing, with no visible signs of diminishing. For that we are both blessed and eternally thankful.

Vera was very fortunate to link herself first with a physician who turned out to be one of the most skilled surgeons in the metropolitan Detroit area (I will not name him, but he certainly knows who he is). Vera and I are very grateful that God sent him to us and for the excellent way in which he performed the surgery to remove the cancerous lump from her breast.

Following the lumpectomy surgery and a series of x-rays and other imaging procedures, we were blessed a second time to be given a very compassionate physician who treated Vera with a regimen of chemotherapy. This was a very challenging experience for all of us. However, this very compassionate oncologist, with the help of a very capable and professional staff, guided Vera through eight very difficult treatments. I am convinced that God also sent her and her wonderful staff our way, and again, we are very thankful for each of them.

I would be remiss if I didn't mention the third step in my wife's treatment, the radiation therapy. This was the portion of the treatment plan that concerned us a great deal. We had heard the horror stories about women being badly scarred and seriously injured with radiation treatment. Again, we were fortunate that God provided us with an excellent and talkative physician who demonstrated a deep concern for us (and I'm sure for all of his patients) and assured us that we would receive the best treatment to be found anywhere. We also were very fortunate to be treated by a highly trained and dedicated staff that was able to treat Vera in a very delicate and compassionate manner; we would like to extend our heartfelt thanks to each of them as well.

Vera got through her treatments successfully, and we turned our attention to growing very old together. In our attempt to become senior citizens, Vera and I have taken on some very wonderful habits: eating highly nutritious food, drinking appropriate amounts of fresh fruit and vegetable juices (mainly organic carrot juice with a splash of natural pomegranate), drinking six to eight glasses of water each day, and getting approximately eight hours of rest each night; we're working on exercising regularly.

I hope you enjoy these next few pages and pray that you are able to take something of value from them. Our deepest prayer is that you will be able to use this information to gain more knowledge or to simply have important information provided in a very casual manner that stimulates you to generate discussion and thoughts about one of the most important parts of your life: your health.

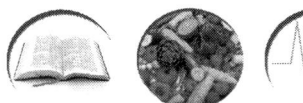

CHAPTER 1

FRUIT

Then God said "I give you every seed-bearing plant on the face of the whole earth and every tree that has fruit with seed in it. They will be yours for food."
—Genesis 1:29 (NIV)

The Creator got it right when he decided to provide humankind with the most important food it would need to sustain the miraculous and holy temple entrusted to each of us, commonly referred to as the body. This scripture is an uncomplicated description and picture of what God created in his likeness and what the body would need for proper nourishment in fulfilling the awesome assignment of ruling over all the earth. Simply put, fruit is one of the most important foods on the planet!

Before informing you of the natural properties and health benefits associated with various fruits, I'll provide you with a small summary concerning this critically important and nutritious food group.

Most fruits are a great source of dietary fiber, which supports digestive health and plays an important role in reducing the risk of colorectal disease and other major health issues; water-rich fruits are especially helpful. Fruit contains valuable minerals, such as potassium, magnesium, iron, phosphorous, calcium, copper, manganese, zinc, and more. Fruit also contains critical health-promoting vitamins, including vitamin

A; B-complex vitamins, including folate, for supporting healthy arteries; vitamins C, D, E, and K, cooperating to improve and sustain health; and a host of antioxidant and anti-inflammatory phytonutrients that prevent cancer-causing free-radical activity in addition to providing other significant health benefits. Together, these nutrients are proven combatants against heart disease; immune dysfunction; nerve and circulatory issues; chronic disease, such as asthma and arthritis; bone and muscle fatigue; blood-sugar imbalance; and many other health disorders. These nutrients act as fighters and protectors on your behalf and are a lightning rod for health and healing.

To realize their powerful nutritional value, the United States Department of Agriculture (USDA) recommends nine servings of fruits and vegetables daily, including four full (1/2 cup) servings of fruit. However, the actual amount required for each person depends on age, gender, level of physical activity, metabolism, and health status. Although fruit and its fiber is important in maintaining blood-sugar balance, large quantities of fruit that have a high sugar content may not be right for a sedentary lifestyle or people who have sugar limitations due to diabetes or other health issues. Elevated levels of glucose in the bloodstream over time can lead to diabetic complications as well as other cardiovascular issues. Talk to your health-care professional as needed concerning the appropriate amounts of this critically important superfood to consume.

Fruit is also a tremendous partner in reducing harsh acidic conditions in the body caused largely by acid-producing foods such as meat, dairy, nuts, corn, wheat, and refined sugars that are heavily consumed in the Standard American Diet. Properly maintaining an alkaline state in the body is vitally important; an overly acidic body is a great environment for debilitating and chronic diseases such as cancer. The kidneys play a major role in buffering and supporting the body's proper pH balance by coordinating, neutralizing, and eliminating excess acid; bones and muscle play a vital role as well. A diet that includes fresh fruits, particularly those containing sufficient amounts of potassium, reduces the strain on the body's acid-reducing components. Decreasing salt intake and staying hydrated with water are also helpful. A little secret: the citric acid in lemon actually has an alkalizing effect in the body. Lemon is regarded as one of the best alkalizing fruits.

Something else you should understand about fruit is the importance of eating it in the morning prior to combining it with other foods; fruit is a natural cleanser. The digestive act sends fruit into the small intestines more quickly than other foods, which assist in providing the morning energy and alertness required to get the body off to a great start. Drinking water first to hydrate from the nighttime resting period and then eating fruit alone on an empty stomach in the morning is the best way to quickly absorb the complete set of nutrients, including the cleansing and healing properties contained in this medical marvel. Consuming other heavy and devitalized foods first in the morning—bacon, donuts, biscuit sandwiches, and the like—following your nighttime fasting period places immediate and ill-considered digestive demands on your body.

As a start, depending on your personal health status and level of activity, choose fresh fruit with appropriate sugar and fiber content; consume what's right for you. Eat your fruit, and if you're still hungry an hour or so later after giving the fruit ample time to assimilate, make another healthy morning food decision—no, not the cinnamon roll with the extra-heavy icing. If you get hungry later in the afternoon between the lunch and dinner hours, fresh fruit is a great refresher and pick-me-up, a much better choice than a caffeine-filled and health-robbing energy drink or sugary candy bar!

By starting with fruit, you give your body the early boost and morning cleanse it requires, and you avoid slowing the early digestive process and inviting its related complications.

Be sure to refrigerate cut and peeled fruit to avoid the risk of foodborne illness. To reduce the amount of pesticides lingering on many fruits, wash all fruit well when eating the skin; purchase organic whenever possible. Also, try to refrain from eating fresh fruits and vegetables at the same time because they digest at different rates; fruits digest quickly, and vegetables digest much slower. Putting them together can rob you of their full nutritional value. Exercise caution in eating fruits with high sugar content at bedtime; the energy derived from the natural sugar may keep you from counting sheep right away. And, of course, follow the advice of your medical professional concerning the amount of fruit you should consume based on your personal health status. For your convenience, each of the fruits discussed in this chapter include total sugar content.

In addressing fruit and blood sugar, glycemic index (GI) information concerning fruit and other food types can be very helpful and is widely available. The GI is a rating scale that reflects how rapidly carbohydrates in food turn to sugar in the blood. Fruits and vegetables tend to have a low to moderate GI. A more recent measure is glycemic load (GL), which measures the amount of carbohydrates in food converting to sugar. Together, the index and load more accurately depict the cumulative effect on blood sugar. An example would be the watermelon. It has a relatively high glycemic index of 72, yet the glycemic load of a medium wedge (286 grams) of watermelon is relatively low (6), which indicates that although there is a rapid conversion (carbohydrate to sugar) rating, there aren't enough carbohydrates in a moderate serving to necessarily have a negative effect on blood sugar. For your convenience, each of the fruits discussed in this chapter includes the GI and GL ratings. Any fruit with a high GI or GL should be eaten either sparingly or in appropriate portions based on health status and consultation with your health-care provider!

Glycemic index: Low = 55 or less; Medium = 56–69; High = 70 and above
Glycemic load: Low = 10 or less; Medium = 11–19; High = 20 and above

Finally, I offer a brief word concerning juicing. Natural fruit juices are excellent for the body's overall health when consumed in moderation. However, fruit juice containing a generous supply of sugar without the natural fiber to regulate blood sugar balance can contribute to an increase in the body's triglyceride levels. The risk increases when combined with the consumption of unhealthy fats. Triglycerides are fats in the blood that can lead to eventual heart disease. Let me be clear: I'm not an opponent of enjoying fresh fruit juice and its related health benefits; I occasionally enjoy a moderate amount of freshly made fruit juice myself. However, regularly consuming larger amounts may impact your health status enough to warrant a discussion with your health-care provider. According to healthy-eating.sfgate.com, the Harvard University School of Public Health recommends no more than a single half-cup daily serving of fruit juice.

Apples

You've heard the old saying "an apple a day keeps the doctor away." Here's why: apples contain phytonutrients (flavonoids) that have several health-promoting and disease-preventing agents, which protect us from chronic diseases such as cancer by binding and arresting free-radical activity. Apples' phytonutrient antioxidant strength can also reduce the oxidation of fats in the bloodstream, significantly reducing the risk of cardiovascular disease and stroke. Studies are showing that the anti-inflammatory phytonutrients in apples play an active role in reducing the risk of asthma. The phytonutrients in apples also combine with their pectin fiber to play a critical role in controlling blood sugar by slowing down carbohydrate digestion, which reduces the release of sugar into the bloodstream. The generous fiber in apples also aids in maintaining a healthy and functional digestive tract through the elimination of waste and cancer-causing toxins from the colon, reducing the risk of colorectal disease and providing relief for the liver in its detoxification efforts.

Apples contain several other health-promoting nutrients, including vitamin A, which reduces the risk of lung and oral-cavity cancers; Vitamin C, a natural antioxidant, which boosts the immune system in protecting the body from cancer causing free-radical cell damage; ample B vitamins; and vitamin K. Apples also contain several vital minerals, including calcium, iron, phosphorous, magnesium, and a great source of potassium for healthy blood pressure. Apples contain an ample supply of chromium, which supports insulin in the proper absorption of glucose into the cells for energy.

It's important to mention that apples should be washed and rinsed thoroughly to limit the amount of harmful pesticides that are often found in apple orchards, and because of a traceable amount of arsenic contained in the seeds, they should not be eaten or included in the juicing process. The skin and flesh of apples, can, however, be combined with other fruits or vegetables in the juicing process. Eat apples with the peel to absorb a large percentage of the antioxidants; buy organic when possible. One medium-sized apple contains 19 grams of sugar, 0.47 grams of protein, 95 calories, and 4.4 grams of dietary fiber; GI: 38/GL: 6.2.

Bananas

Bananas are a fruit containing important phytochemicals in the form of carotene, which actively controls cell-damaging free radicals. Bananas contain a favorable amount of protein for building and repairing tissue and supporting the immune system. Bananas also contain a significant supply of fiber for regulating the rate of digestion to balance blood sugar and for providing support to maintain the healthy bacteria in the colon, which contributes to the overall health of the digestive system.

Bananas have an ample amount of important minerals, including a generous supply of potassium for maintaining proper water balance in the blood and regulating heart rate and blood pressure, manganese for facilitating calcium absorption and proper thyroid function, magnesium and calcium for healthy bone structure, and iron for transporting oxygen to cells and tissues. Other important minerals found in bananas support healthy cell function throughout the body, heal wounds, and provide antioxidant support. A medium-sized fresh banana contains an assortment of B vitamins, including B6 for new cell development and other B vitamins for proper muscle and nervous system function; vitamin C for reducing the risk of infection; vitamin E for immune system health and healthy hair; and vitamin K for retaining minerals in the bone and facilitating proper blood clotting.

Bananas should be eaten fully ripened to absorb all the vital nutrients and their related health benefits. Refrigeration may prevent the ripening process; however, it's OK to refrigerate and store fully ripe bananas in a plastic bag (to reduce darkening) for an extra one or two days of enjoyment. One medium banana contains 14 grams of sugar, 1.29 grams of protein, 105 calories, 422 milligrams of potassium, and 3.1 grams of dietary fiber; GI: 62/GL: 12.2.

Oranges

Oranges are low in calories, contain no cholesterol, and are an excellent source of pectin fiber, which serves to properly and safely move waste and toxins through the digestive tract, reducing the risk of colorectal disease and constipation. Oranges have a rich supply of phytonutrients that significantly reduces the severity of inflammatory conditions such as asthma and rheumatoid arthritis and prevents the oxidation or hardening of cholesterol, which can be caused by free-radical activity.

As you might expect, oranges contain a generous supply of vitamin C, a primary antioxidant that fights infection and free-radical development to reduce the risk of cellular DNA damage; vitamin C is one of the best defenders against cancer-causing cell mutation. Oranges also have a nice supply of vitamin A for growing and repairing tissue and vigorously reducing the risk of lung and oral cancer; B vitamins for developing new cells and strengthening blood vessels; and vitamin E for supporting a healthy immune system and aiding normal growth and development. Oranges also contain a variety of minerals including calcium for reducing the risk of osteoporosis, copper for red blood cell formation, iron for transporting oxygen to tissues and cells, magnesium for bone mineralization, and zinc for healthy male reproduction.

The potassium, vitamin C, carotenoids, and flavonoids found in fresh oranges, with their combined antioxidant strength, add greater protection to the cardiovascular system. According to the George Mateljan Foundation, a major study discovered that an extra daily serving of citrus fruit can reduce the risk of stroke by 19 percent. One medium orange contains 13 grams of sugar, 1.23 grams of protein, 62 calories, 237 milligrams of potassium, and 3.1 grams of dietary fiber; GI: 43/GL: 4.

Pineapples

Pineapples contain important phytonutrients such as beta-carotene, which provides invaluable support for the prevention of cell and tissue damage. Fiber is present and plays a significant role in increasing colon health and balancing blood sugar. Pineapples contain an enzyme called bromelain, which contributes to the effective breakdown and digestion of protein. Also, the bromelain and papain enzymes in pineapple are fierce enemies of parasite activity in the digestive tract.

Pineapples are a rich source of vitamin C, which stands guard against the development of free radicals in the body, which reduces the risk of chronic disease such as cancer and effectively minimizes the growth of infection. The vitamin C contained in fresh pineapples is a great partner in fighting the inflammatory and painful conditions of osteoarthritis and rheumatoid arthritis. Vitamin A, B vitamins, and vitamin K are all present to provide active protection for the lungs, eyes, muscles, nerves, and arteries. Pineapples also contain a rich supply of the trace mineral manganese for facilitating the absorption of calcium and enabling the body to properly utilize its supply of antioxidants; copper for aiding the absorption of iron; and magnesium, potassium, phosphorous, selenium, and zinc to provide bone protection, strengthen blood vessels, and provide antioxidant support.

Excessive amounts of bromelain reportedly can cause skin rashes and diarrhea and can negatively interact with some medications, including antibiotics and blood thinners; talk to your health-care professional as appropriate. Taking three years to mature, one cup of pineapple contains 16 grams of sugar, 0.89 grams of protein, 82 calories, and 2.3 grams of dietary fiber; GI: 66/GL: 6.

Plums

One of the major benefits of plums is that they help to regulate smooth functioning of the digestive tract, helping to relieve constipation. Fresh plums are a moderate source of vitamin A, vitamin C, and beta-carotene. Vitamin A is essential for healthy eyesight and recently has been shown to provide protection from lung and oral cancers. Vitamin C and beta-carotene have superior antioxidant nutrients to fight against chronic diseases such as cancer, asthma, and arthritis. Plums also contain several other health-promoting flavonoid phytonutrients.

Plums contain an ample amount of potassium, which contributes significantly to resilient arteries and a healthy cardiovascular system, and iron, which is necessary for transporting oxygen to cells and tissues and red blood cell formation and function. One small plum contains 7 grams of sugar, 0.5 grams of protein, 30 calories, and 1 gram of dietary fiber; GI: 24/GL: 2.

Peaches

Peaches are very similar to plums in their vitamin and mineral makeup; they contain vitamin A, vitamin C, beta-carotene, flavonoids, potassium, iron, and other vital nutrients, all working harmoniously together to support and increase health. Like plums, peaches contain vitamin K, which is required for proper clotting of blood, and vitamins E and B5, both of which are required for normal growth and development.

Peaches are very sweet yet low in calories and can be used in a weight-control plan to replace treats containing processed sugar. According to research scientist Dr. Luis Cisneros-Zevallos, an associate professor at Texas A&M University, stone fruits such as peaches, plums, and nectarines contain phytochemicals that have antiobesity, antidiabetic, and anti-inflammatory properties in different cell lines and can be effective in fighting metabolic syndrome. One medium peach contains 13 grams of sugar, 1.36 grams of protein, 58 calories, and 2.2 grams of dietary fiber; GI: 28/GL: 5.

Blueberries

Blueberries are one of the few fruits native to North America. Information provided by The World's Healthiest Foods at www.whfoods.com indicates there is evidence that blueberries can have positive effects on memory. A study involving older adults strongly reflected an improvement in cognitive function when fed a generous amount of fresh-squeezed blueberry juice. Blueberries are well known for maintaining neurological health and cognitive ability.

Blueberries contain several critical vitamins and minerals, and it's important to note that organically grown blueberries have been discovered to have a higher amount of antioxidants than those grown conventionally. A further review of the information at www.whfoods.com reveals that blueberries contain one of the highest antioxidant capacities among all fruits and are shown to add strength and protection in several body systems, including the cardiovascular, nervous, and digestive systems, in addition to promoting muscular health. According to Dr. Joseph Mercola, blueberries are champions for increasing and maintaining the good bacteria in the colon, protecting the colon from inflammation causing toxins. There is plenty of information to support the fact that blueberries, which rank low in the glycemic index, are great for regulating blood sugar.

The rich level of phytonutrients in blueberries has an increasing correlation to anticancer benefits and improved eye health. Studies have also shown that blueberries lose very few of their nutrient properties when frozen for later consumption. Due to the use of pesticides, be sure to wash and rinse conventionally grown blueberries—and all berries—thoroughly. One cup of blueberries contains 15 grams of sugar, 1.1 grams of protein, 84 calories, and 3.6 grams of dietary fiber; GI: 40/GL: 6.

Strawberries

Strawberries are one of the most nutritious low-calorie foods. Filled with super antioxidant capabilities, they are a good source of the minerals manganese and potassium. A cup of fresh strawberries contains more vitamin C than a medium-sized orange, which explains strawberries' excellent antioxidant and anti-inflammatory benefits. The excellent phytonutrient power of strawberries is a major reason they're highly recommended for maintaining a healthy immune system in the fight against various forms of cancer, including breast, colon, and cervical cancers, while simultaneously decreasing the oxidation of fats in our blood vessels, providing support for a healthy cardiovascular system. Research has also revealed that strawberries are a tremendous ally in regulating proper blood-sugar levels.

To realize the potent strength of the antioxidant and anti-inflammatory properties contained in berries, many health experts recommend including a one-cup serving at least three times a week. Because of their perishable nature, strawberries lose their antioxidant power and vitamins quickly; you'll want to refrigerate and consume them within a couple of days of purchase if possible. Freeze them whole when necessary and purchase organic whenever possible. One cup of fresh strawberries contains 7 grams of sugar, 0.96 grams of protein, 46 calories, and 2.9 grams of dietary fiber; GI: 40/GL: 3.6.

Grapes

Grapes contain powerful antioxidant flavonoids that greatly reduce the damage and effects of free radicals. These antioxidants can prevent the oxidation of cholesterol, reducing the risk of blood-clogging cardiovascular complications. Grapes also aid in decreasing further risk within the cardiovascular system by supplying nitric oxide in the blood, which improves blood flow. Due to the high level of water grapes contain, they are a great cleanser helping to remove acid buildup and filtering dangerous toxins from the blood, which relieves stress on the kidneys and liver.

The dietary fiber in grapes promotes blood-sugar balance, has a positive effect on insulin regulation, and aids in relieving constipation by pushing foods through the digestive tract; significantly benefitting colon health. The vitamins in grapes, particularly vitamin C, support and boost the body's immune system. The combination of the minerals iron, copper, and manganese contribute significantly to maintaining bone health and delivering oxygen for healthy cell function throughout the body. The phytonutrients and water content in grapes are therapeutic in combating the chronic effects of asthma. Research indicates that the phytonutrients in grapes have been shown to combat infection, multiple forms of cancer, and retinal disease; the phytonutrient resveratrol, in red grapes, reportedly has beneficial effects on Alzheimer's disease.

Due to the heavy use of pesticides in grape crops, it's better to consume organic grapes when possible. One cup of grapes contains 23 grams of sugar, 1.09 grams of protein, 104 calories, and 1.4 grams of dietary fiber; GI: 59/GL: 11.

Watermelon

As its name implies, watermelon is an excellent hydrating food originating in Africa. Watermelon is rich in two powerful antioxidants, vitamins A and C, and has an abundant supply of the antioxidant phytonutrient lycopene, a well-publicized prostate-cancer fighter.

Watermelon's lycopene content is superior to that found in fresh tomatoes. In addition to providing defense against lung and oral-cavity cancer and growing and repairing tissue, the rich vitamin A content aids in providing properties to the colon lining that facilitate the release of waste from the colon, reducing the risk of colorectal disease. Vitamin C promotes a healthy and active immune system to eradicate free-radical activity before it starts, reducing the risk of cancer-causing DNA damage.

Watermelon is composed of mostly water at 92 percent but contains an ample supply of potassium, which promotes soft and resilient arteries and regulates blood pressure and heart rate. Watermelon further supports heart health by supplying nitric oxide to the blood, improving blood flow. It's better to eat fully ripened fresh watermelon to gain its full health benefits.

The white seeds in seedless watermelons are actually empty seed coverings. One medium wedge of watermelon contains 18 grams of sugar, 1.74 grams of protein, 86 calories, and 1.1 grams of dietary fiber; GI: 72/GL: 6.

Lemons

A powerful antioxidant and phytonutrient-rich citrus fruit, lemons are loaded with vitamin C and potassium. Lemons treat infection and kill germs with their antiseptic qualities, soothe respiratory disorders, strengthen the immune system, combat chronic disease such as cancer, prevent the formation of kidney stones, control high blood pressure, flush toxins from the body, and aid in detoxifying and energizing the liver. Juice from half a lemon with water is a great cleanser to start your day. One medium lemon contains 2 grams of sugar, 0.92 grams of protein, 24 calories, and 2.4 grams of dietary fiber; GI: Low/GL: 3.

Limes

Limes are a citrus fruit with great antioxidants and several health benefits, according to www.organicfacts.net. Their benefits include nourishing skin, aiding digestion, relieving constipation, regulating blood sugar, reducing toxins for joint health, and improving urinary tract issues. Limes contain more vitamin A and less vitamin C than lemons, but have cleansing qualities similar to those of lemons. The limes' fame increased when discovered as a cure for scurvy, an infectious disease amongst British sailors on extended voyage assignments. A single lime contains 20 calories, 1 gram of sugar, and 2 grams of fiber.

Cherries

A fruit bursting with health benefits and nutritional properties, cherries provide melatonin, which lowers the body temperature and calms the nervous system to promote sound sleep. Cherries support a healthy cardiovascular system with their ample supply of potassium.

The phytonutrients found in cherries contain properties that protect the body from free radicals and their cumulative capacity to create cell and tissue damage. The anti-inflammatory phytonutrients in tart cherries and their juice reportedly reduce incidents and the related pain of arthritis and gout attacks, and also soothe muscle pain. Cherries also contain vitamin C for increasing immune health and a moderate supply of phosphorous to strengthen bones and teeth. One cup of fresh cherries contains 20 grams of sugar, 1.46 grams of protein, 87 calories, and 2.9 grams of dietary fiber; GI: 22/GL: 7.

Pears

Pears contain an excellent amount of water-soluble pectin fiber, which helps to eliminate fatty substances from the digestive tract. Pears also serve to properly move waste and toxins through the digestive tract and colon; reducing the risk of colorectal disease and constipation.

Pears contain an ample amount of minerals, including potassium, phosphorous, and magnesium, as well as vitamin A, B-complex vitamins, and vitamin C, which also shields the body from the harmful effects of cancer-causing free radicals. It's important to note that the majority of the pear's antioxidant and anti-inflammatory phytonutrients and half of its dietary fiber reside in the skin. According to www.whfoods.com, the healthy flavonoid antioxidant strength of pears has been shown to reduce the risk of type 2 diabetes, especially in women.

Pears are very digestible and have a very low allergic response. One medium pear contains 17 grams of sugar, 0.68 grams of protein, 103 calories, and 5.5 grams of dietary fiber; GI: 38/GL: 6.

Avocado

This fruit originated in Mexico and, due to its appearance, is commonly referred to as "alligator pears." The avocado's skin helps protect the fruit from pesticides. Avocados contain polyunsaturated omega 3 fatty acids as well as monounsaturated fatty acid, which can be burned easily for energy. The majority of the calories in avocados are in their fatty acid. They're also quite low in cholesterol.

Avocados have a very generous supply of potassium that almost doubles the amount found in bananas to regulate blood pressure, heart rate, and electrolyte balance. Like bananas, they continue to ripen after harvest. Avocados contain other important minerals, including phosphorous, calcium, and copper working together to strengthen bone density, and a very generous supply of dietary fiber to enhance a healthy digestive tract and colon. Avocados contain several vitamins, including vitamins B, C, E, and K. Avocado also slows the breakdown of food into usable sugar, thereby increasing the regulation of blood sugar. Avocados are low in sugar and contain several phytonutrients that nourish the eyes, hair, and skin; support heart and liver health; aid in nutrient absorption; and combat the cancer-causing effects of free radicals. These phytonutrients also combine with avocado's omega 3 fatty acids to reduce inflammation and pain commonly associated with arthritis.

It is important to note that avocados have been known to trigger migraine conditions. Although avocados are healthy, if you're not burning their higher calorie and fat content efficiently, you may want to adjust your consumption of them accordingly. A medium-sized avocado contains 1 gram of sugar, 4.02 grams of protein, 22.5 grams of fat, 322 calories, 700 milligrams of potassium, and 13.5 grams of dietary fiber; GI: Low/GL: 4.

Papaya

Papaya is a rich source of vitamins, minerals, and phytonutrients. Papaya is one of the highest sources of vitamin C, containing even more than oranges, and provides tremendous health benefits to the body's immune system. Papaya also contains a sizable amount of vitamin A, which is essential for night vision, growth and repair of body tissue, and combating lung and oral cancers. The digestive enzyme in papaya, papain, helps to restore balance in the digestive tract and is known to be unwelcoming to intestinal parasites.

This amazing fruit also contains plenty of potassium to support cardiovascular health. Papaya contains several phytonutrients, including lycopene, an antioxidant that is heavily associated with preventing prostate and other cancers and reducing the risk of chronic diseases such as asthma. Papaya is also known to have positive health effects in relation to diabetes by lowering blood sugar, and sufficient dietary fiber to improve digestion and protect the colon from toxins. One cup of cubed, fresh papaya contains 11 grams of sugar, 0.85 grams of protein, 55 calories, and 2.5 grams of dietary fiber; GI: 60/GL: 10.

Pomegranate

This delicious fruit originated in the Iraq and Iran regions and contains a generous amount of potassium, which regulates heart rate and muscle functions, and smoothes arteries for improved blood circulation. Pomegranate also contains an ample amount of vitamin C, which boosts the body's immune function; several other key vitamins, including B5, E, and K; and critical minerals, such as copper and manganese, which are important contributors to bone density. Also included in this amazing fruit is an ample supply of dietary fiber to support a healthy digestive tract.

A key health benefit is the number of antioxidants within the pomegranate, which neutralize free radicals in the body, thereby reducing cell and tissue damage. Studies have shown that the phytonutrient properties in the fruit and peel play a significant role in reducing the risk of breast, lung, and prostate cancer. In addition to several powerful antioxidants, pomegranates contain antitumor and antiviral nutrients, which support the fight against chronic disease and improve dental and oral health.

You can feel free to eat only the juicy arils, which surround the seeds, or both—your choice. You may also choose to press the arils and seeds for the juice. However, the processing of commercial no-sugar-added, fresh-pressed pomegranate juice leaves the peel intact during the pressing process, such that this juice contains a higher level of antioxidant health benefits; it's also great for adding a splash of flavor to water. Because of the high sugar and calories in the pomegranate, eat sparingly or in appropriate portions based on your health status. One fresh pomegranate contains 39 grams of sugar, 4.71 grams of protein, 234 calories, and 11.3 grams of dietary fiber. GI: 67/GL: 18.

Kiwifruit

This fruit is native to China. It was originally called the Chinese gooseberry, and then later harvested in New Zealand and named after New Zealand's kiwi bird. Kiwis are small but mighty and are a good source of vitamins C, K, and folate. Minerals include potassium for a healthy heart and blood pressure; phosphorous, calcium, and magnesium combine to sustain healthy bones. The vitamin C content alone is more than oranges in a relative size comparison, and as you well know, vitamin C is an important cog in driving a robust immune system.

This small fruit and its phytonutrient strength can handle big jobs such as protecting DNA in the cells from oxidation and can have a positive impact on inflammatory diseases, such as osteoarthritis, rheumatoid arthritis, and complications associated with asthma. Kiwi contains ample fiber to support digestive health, including the removal of dangerous toxins in the colon, and to regulate blood-sugar levels. One medium kiwi contains 6 grams of sugar, 0.79 grams of protein, 42 calories, and 2.1 grams of dietary fiber; GI: 53/GL: 4.

Dried Fruit

Dried fruit contains very little water following natural sun drying or mechanical drying, and it takes approximately three to four pounds of fresh fruit to create a single pound of dried fruit. Dried fruits generally contain higher fiber content, and in an even weight comparison, dried fruit contains more calories, vitamins, minerals, and phytonutrients than its fresh siblings. Dried fruits are rich in iron, which is required for transporting oxygen to cells and tissues and building red blood cells.

Some dried fruits have more sugar and calories than others, but all have enough of both to warrant monitoring the amount you consume. In some instances, dried fruits, especially cherries and cranberries, have added sugar, which makes it doubly important to monitor your intake. Don't confuse dried fruit with snack foods that you enjoy in larger quantities; you'll likely have trouble fastening your jeans. Dried fruit is also pretty sticky and can create cavities sooner than normal. Stay away from dried fruit treated with preserving agents such as sulphur dioxide; sulphur dioxide can have a negative respiratory effect on individuals with asthma.

Many of the dried fruits are rated low to moderate on the glycemic index chart, but be cautious not to overconsume. Raisins have a high glycemic load and account for almost half of the dried fruit sold; one 1.5-ounce box of raisins contains 25 grams of sugar, 1.32 grams of protein, 129 calories, 322 milligrams of potassium, and 1.6 grams of dietary fiber; GI: 64/GL: 20.5.

Summary
As stated earlier, the highlighted fruits are those most commonly consumed and consequently merited the highest consideration for discussion. I hope your favorites were included. You can review the additional resource pages for the names of online sites that contain several other fruits and their related health benefits.

Food for Thought:

- Eat fruit in the morning, following your initial water intake.
- Eat fruits and their natural sugar in proportion to your health status and activity; four half-cup daily servings of fresh fruit are recommended; fruit juice should be limited to 1/2-cup daily.

- Select fruits that contain the vitamin, mineral, and fiber combination that's right for you.
- For increased nutrient value, purchase fresh fruits from trusted local farms or stores that supply local farm produce when available.
- Exercise caution in overconsuming fresh or commercial fruit juices; they can increase triglyceride (fat in blood) levels.
- Refrain from eating whole fruits and vegetables at the same time due to their different rates of digestion and the possibility that the fruit's nutrition may be compromised.
- It's OK to juice fruits and vegetables together; their digestion is much quicker than when you eat whole fruits and vegetables together.
- Apples contain an ample supply of chromium, which supports insulin in the proper absorption of glucose into the cells for energy; they're also great for moving toxins safely through the digestive tract and colon.
- Lemons are great for flushing toxins from the body and aid in detoxifying and energizing the liver.
- The bromelain and papain enzymes in pineapple are fierce enemies of parasite activity in the digestive tract.
- The anti-inflammatory phytonutrients in tart cherries and their juice reportedly reduce incidents and the related pain of arthritis and gout attacks, and also soothe muscle pain.
- The phytonutrients and water content in grapes are therapeutic in combating the chronic effects of asthma.
- Blueberries are great for maintaining neurological health and cognitive ability.
- Organic berries have a higher antioxidant capacity than those grown conventionally, which is great in fighting chronic diseases.
- Any fruit with a high glycemic index or glycemic load should be eaten either sparingly or in proper portions based on your health status; talk to your health-care provider.

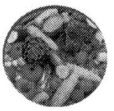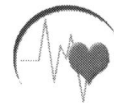

CHAPTER 2

VEGETABLES

"Daniel then said to the guard whom the chief official had appointed over Daniel, Hananiah, Mishael, and Azariah, 'Please test your servants for ten days: Give us nothing but vegetables to eat and water to drink. Then compare our appearance with that of the young men who eat the royal food, and treat your servants in accordance with what you see.' So he agreed to this and tested them for ten days. At the end of the ten days they looked healthier and better nourished than any of the young men who ate the royal food."
—DANIEL 1:11–15 (NIV)

You've heard the old adage, "The more things change, the more they stay the same." The profound discovery Daniel offered thousands of years ago concerning the health effects of vegetables is as important today as it was when he first spoke it. I'm far from being a rocket scientist; however, it's clear to me that Daniel had very keen insight and wisdom at such a young age. Like Daniel, our goal is to be healthy. Say it with me three times—healthy, healthy, healthy!

Now that you're properly hypnotized, let's talk a little about vegetables and their important nutritional value and related health benefits. First of all, as you might expect, vegetables are low in calories and fats and are a storehouse of many vital nutrients such as dietary fiber for maintaining a healthy digestive system and for reducing the risk of colorectal disease, regulating blood sugar, and reducing cholesterol in the blood in support of overall heart health. Vegetables are much lower in natural sugar content when compared to fruit. Eating nine servings of fruits and vegetables daily, including five full (1/2-cup) servings of vegetables, is recommended.

Vegetables can easily be designated as a building and strengthening food with their rich source of bone-strengthening minerals, including calcium and magnesium, largely found in green leafy vegetables. Other minerals commonly found in vegetables include potassium for regulating heart rate and blood pressure and maintaining fluid balance in support of cell integrity; iron for aiding in transporting oxygen to organs and tissues. There's also a combination of phosphorous, copper, and zinc for strengthening bones, forming red blood cells, and healing wounds; and many more.

Also, as you might expect, vegetables contain an abundant supply of vitamins, including vitamin A for maintaining eye health, providing protection against lung and oral-cavity cancers, and growing and repairing damaged body tissue; a host of B vitamins, which are important for energy metabolism, proper nerve function, digestion of carbohydrates, protein metabolism, normal growth and development, and other healthy bodily functions; folate, also a B vitamin, which helps to form red blood cells and provides protection for an unborn fetus; vitamin C for increasing the health of the immune system to reduce the risk of cellular DNA damage and chronic disease and infection; vitamin E, which acts as an antioxidant to prevent cell damage and helps to maintain healthy skin and hair; and Vitamin K, which adds to the "building and strengthening" mantra due to its ability to retain minerals inside the bone and actively regulates blood calcium levels to decrease the hardening of arteries.

As you well know, vegetables come in a wide array of rich colors. A host of phytonutrients reside in these richly colored vegetables (some are discussed later in the book). However, the book would not be complete without the mention of the great alkalizing, phytochemical chlorophyll, which provides the pigment in green vegetables, and together with enriching sunlight stored in plants, provides several health and nutritional benefits. Chlorophyll heals wounds; boosts the immune system; forms new red blood cells; increases oxygen capacity in the blood; and cleanses the blood of toxins and metals, providing significant support to the liver. Chlorophyll adds protection to the colon from carcinogenic agents in meat grilled and charred at high temperatures, and aids in reducing arthritic inflammation in the body.

Make sure you purchase healthy-looking fresh vegetables. Vegetables like fruit often have a brief shelf life and lose their vital health benefits in a short period of time. Buy fresh and eat fresh as often as possible. Many vegetables are treated with several pesticides, many of which are carcinogenic agents that have overall devastating effects on the body, including damage to the immune and nervous systems. Be sure to wash all vegetables very carefully, especially those that are not peeled or scraped; purchase organic whenever possible. Studies have discovered that eating the appropriate amount of vegetables in your minimum servings of fresh fruits and vegetables protects the body from stroke, arthritis, and several other debilitating and chronic diseases. Raw or lightly steamed, vegetables provide a high level of nutritional value; don't cook the life out of them!

Like fruit, the vast majority of vegetables are alkaline-forming and has similar nutritional properties. However, it's important to point out again that vegetables and fruits are very different in terms of the time it takes to digest them. Fruit is digested very quickly through the stomach and into the intestine, while vegetables take a longer period of time to digest. If you eat them together, just know that the fruit can be held in the stomach far longer than usual and ultimately may not provide a full complement of nutrients as it would if eaten alone.

A multitude of different vegetables are grown and imported from around the world. Some of the more common vegetables consumed on a regular basis are featured. The vegetable nutrient profile is included at the end of each description, including the glycemic load (GL), which measures the amount of carbohydrate in food converting to sugar and its effect on blood sugar.

Glycemic Load: Low = 10 or less; Medium = 11–19; High = 20 and above

Before reviewing each vegetable below, it's important to offer a word about vegetable juice. As part of an intensive study, the National Institute of Health concluded that one to two cups of vegetable juice daily is an acceptable way for healthy adults to increase their consumption of vegetables; five full (½-cup) servings of vegetables is recommended. The specific amount of juice consumed can be applied to the recommended daily servings of vegetables. The use of low sodium or sodium free vegetables for juicing would be a better choice for overall health. According to the online site, www.fruitsandveggiesmorematters.org, low sodium or sodium free vegetables include bell pepper, broccoli, carrots, celery, cucumbers (sodium free), tomatoes (very low sodium), and several other vegetables. Talk to your health-care provider concerning the use of vegetable juice as a substitute for regular vegetable consumption.

Carrots

Carrot is a root vegetable, the underground root of a plant used as a vegetable food. Carrots are low in calories and contain no cholesterol. As you know, carrots are crunchy, have plenty of snap, and are commonly brilliant orange in color; there are other varietal colors. Carrots are very rich in beta-carotene (a five-star general) and vitamin A, combining to supply a tremendous amount of antioxidant nutrition and firepower in the battle against free-radical damage, the major cause of several forms of cancer. The rich source of vitamin A in carrots promotes growth and repair of body tissue; bone formation; and healthy eyes, skin, and hair; and more recently has been reported to stand guard against lung and oral cancer. Carrots also contain vitamin C, another powerful antioxidant, and a complement of B vitamins, including B5 (pantothenic acid), important for proper growth and development.

Carrots are also home to several important minerals, including potassium to regulate heart beat and blood pressure, and calcium and phosphorous working together to strengthen bones and teeth. Carrots contain plenty of fiber to aid the health of the digestive system and the regulation of blood sugar.

Carrots should be scrubbed and rinsed, and enjoyed raw as a snack, lightly steamed as part of a meal, or as a fresh juice; carrots can be juiced in combination with other vegetables or fruit. Carrots and its juice are well known for being a cleansing agent for the liver and for removing harmful metals, such as aluminum, from the fatty tissue in the body, which can reduce the risk of neurodegenerative disorders such as Alzheimer's disease. Carrots can be stored up to two to three weeks when properly refrigerated. You can visit the carrot museum online to learn much more about additional health benefits. One medium carrot contains 25 calories, 2 grams of fiber, 3 grams of sugar, and 1 gram of protein; GL: 2.

Cucumbers

Cucumbers, also considered a fruit, are a vine plant belonging to the squash and melon family and are composed of largely water at 92 percent. Cucumbers are refreshing and contain an ample amount of the electrolyte minerals potassium and magnesium, which together contribute significantly to the control of blood pressure, heart rate, and blood circulation, and also contain the trace mineral silica, which contributes to the healthy growth and maintenance of connective tissue. Cucumbers contain dietary fiber, which helps to eliminate toxins from the body and balance blood sugar. Cucumbers provide additional support leveling blood sugar with the aid of a specific hormone that assists the pancreas in producing insulin. Cucumbers are very low in calories and contain no cholesterol, sodium, or saturated fats, which support healthy weight goals.

Cucumbers contain important phytonutrients such as carotene; vitamins C and A, which protect against inflammation and free-radical damage to cells and tissue; and vitamin K, which is important in proper blood clotting and maintaining bone health. According to The World's Healthiest Foods at www.whfood.com, the lignan phytonutrients contained in cucumbers have the ability to reduce the risk of estrogen-related cancers, such as cancers of the breast, ovaries, uterus, and prostate. The high water content aids in keeping skin moist and soft, and can provide a cooling affect for acid reflux by increasing the pH balance in the stomach. The water and fiber in cucumbers can relieve constipation and prevent the development of kidney stones, and also reduce inflammatory issues such as gout, arthritis, and asthma caused by the buildup of uric acid; meat products, alcoholic beverages, and refined sugar are some of the main contributors to uric acid buildup.

If eating the skin, which contains an ample amount of vitamin C, be sure to wash it thoroughly due to the wax covering and pesticide load. Cucumbers make a very refreshing juice and mix well with other nutrient-rich vegetables. Half a cup of sliced cucumbers contains 8 calories, 0.3 grams fiber, 1 gram of sugar, and 0.34 grams of protein; GL: 1.

Tomatoes

The tomato, also considered a fruit, is native to Central America and belongs to the nightshade family of vegetables that includes potatoes, eggplant, bell peppers, and various hot peppers, including cayenne and jalapeno. Tomatoes are low in calories and fat, and contain no cholesterol. Tomatoes are home to a host of vitamins, minerals, and phytonutrients. A popular antioxidant phytochemical, lycopene, receives a lot of attention relative to its strength to battle cell and tissue damaging free radicals, and plays a major role in the protection against prostate, breast, cervical, colon, and other cancers. Vitamin A is present in tomatoes, which guards against lung and oral cancers, repairs damaged tissue, and supports healthy vision, including night vision. Vitamin C, a powerful antioxidant, reduces the risk of cellular DNA damage, while at the same time fighting infection and sustaining a robust immune system.

Tomatoes are also rich in minerals, such as potassium, which regulates blood pressure and heart rate and maintains proper water balance in the blood; and magnesium, phosphorous, calcium, and copper, which support and sustain healthy bones. According to the website Organic Facts at www.organicfacts.net, regular consumption of tomatoes has been shown to reduce LDL (bad) cholesterol and triglycerides in the blood, minimizing fat deposits in the blood vessels. Tomatoes contain a significant supply of water and fiber, which supports digestive health, and at the same time serves as a diuretic, stimulating the release of urine to expel toxins, salt, and uric acid from the body; the combined effects reduce incidents of urinary tract infections.

Wash and rinse tomatoes thoroughly due to various pesticides used in the conventional growing process; organic tomatoes are better and have been discovered to have a higher level of phytonutrients than those grown conventionally. Select fully ripened tomatoes for full nutrient value. Studies also indicate that lycopene content is more intense in tomato sauces; great for prostate protection and health. Individuals challenged with arthritic conditions may want to talk to their health-care professional concerning the consumption of vegetables in the nightshade family. One medium tomato contains 22 calories, 2.9 grams of fiber, 3 grams of sugar, 292 milligrams of potassium, and 1.08 grams of protein; GL: 2.

Broccoli

Broccoli is a vegetable belonging to the cruciferous family, which includes cabbage, cauliflower, brussels sprouts, and other vegetables. The floret portion of broccoli contains important phytonutrients that contribute significantly to improving health and disease prevention, including the elimination of dangerous toxins from the body. Broccoli contains a small amount of omega-3 fatty acids that works with broccoli's phytonutrients to neutralize chronic inflammation. Broccoli is low in calories; contains no fat; is an excellent source of vitamins, minerals, and dietary fiber; and has significant antioxidant strength, which aids in shielding the body from several cancers, including cancers of the breast, colon, prostate, pancreas, and bladder; can also breakdown estrogen for elimination from the body. Dietary fiber is present to reduce cholesterol levels in the blood and contribute to a healthy stomach and digestive tract.

Broccoli contains an ample amount of vitamin A, which acts as an antioxidant by providing multiple components of protection for the health of the eyes and skin and by providing protection against cancers of the lungs and oral cavity; several B vitamins, that work together to provide health to the nervous system and improve artery health and blood circulation; a generous supply of vitamin C, which engages and supports a robust immune system and stands guard against cancer-causing free-radical activity; and vitamin K, which promotes normal blood clotting and regulates blood calcium to reduce the risk of artery hardening (calcification). Broccoli also contains several important minerals, including potassium for heart health; and phosphorous, magnesium, calcium, and copper for healthy bones.

Broccoli may affect blood-thinning medications and individuals with thyroid and sensitive digestive tract health issues; consult your health-care professional concerning this food if any of these applies to you. One cup of chopped broccoli contains 31 calories, 2 grams of fiber, 2 grams of sugar, and 3 grams of protein; GL: 3.

Cabbage

Cabbage belongs to the cruciferous family of vegetables and comes in several varieties, such as green, red, bok choy, napa, and savoy. Cabbage is rich in phytonutrient antioxidants and is very low in fat and calories; red cabbage has a significantly higher antioxidant value. The phytonutrients in cabbage are well known to stand guard against the damaging effects of cell and tissue damage caused by oxidizing free radicals and is excellent in protecting the body from several cancers, including cancers of the breast, colon, prostate, pancreas, and bladder; can also breakdown estrogen for elimination from the body. Cabbage is highly regarded as a brain food and a proponent in reducing the effects of Alzheimer's disease. Its anti-inflammatory qualities assist in the removal of uric acid and other toxins from the body, which reduces the risk and effects of inflammatory health issues such as arthritis and gout.

Fresh cabbage contains several important vitamins and minerals that provide a variety of health benefits. Cabbage contains an ample supply of vitamin C to support a healthy immune system in the fight against infectious disease and free-radical activity; B-complex vitamins, which support normal functioning of the nervous system; vitamin E for healthy eyes and skin; and vitamin K for proper blood clotting, regulation of blood calcium, and protection against osteoporosis. Cabbage also contains multiple mineral resources, including potassium, a vasodilator that improves blood flow by dilating blood vessels for healthy heart function, as well as providing fluid and electrolyte balance; phosphorous, magnesium, and calcium for bone strength; and smaller amounts of other important minerals that support healthy red blood cell formation and other essential functions. The high fiber content in cabbage aids in moving food through the digestive tract, significantly contributing to the reduction of constipation, and its sulphur content reduces the risk and severity of ulcers in support of stomach health.

To absorb these health-supporting vital nutrients, cabbage should be eaten raw or lightly steamed, which aids in absorbing the cholesterol-lowering benefit. Be sure to wash and rinse cabbage to remove the pesticides used in the conventional growing process. Cabbage may interfere with blood-thinning medications and may also affect individuals with thyroid and sensitive digestive tract health issues; talk to your health-care professional concerning this food if these apply to you. One cup of shredded cabbage contains 17 calories, 2 grams of fiber, 2 grams of sugar, and 1 gram of protein; GL: 1.

Celery

Celery is a very low-calorie plant food and contains a significant amount of dietary fiber, contributing to a healthy digestive tract and colon health. Celery is a source of important vitamins, including vitamins A, B, C, E, and K. Celery is also home to important minerals such as potassium for maintaining blood pressure, heart rate, and fluid levels in the body; and phosphorous, magnesium, calcium, and copper for healthy bones and teeth.

Celery contains several phytochemical compounds that reduce the effects of inflammatory diseases such as arthritis and gout, offering a nourishing treatment to joints and their tissue. The powerful antioxidants in celery lower the effectiveness of carcinogens, significantly reducing the risk of various cancers, specifically breast cancer. According to the George Mateljan Foundation, celery can provide protection to the liver and the digestive tract from cancer-causing toxins created largely by the consumption of fried foods.

Celery acts as a cleansing diuretic to remove excess water, uric acid, and harmful toxins from the body, which reduces the risk of urinary tract infections and, in the process, can improve certain bladder and kidney conditions. Celery actively promotes the release of bile juices, which contributes to the lowering of blood cholesterol.

Wash and rinse celery thoroughly due to pesticide residues; consume organic whenever possible. The highest level of nutrition occurs when eaten raw or lightly steamed with other vegetables. Celery may impact individuals who have certain allergies; talk to your health-care professional if this is a concern. One cup of chopped celery contains 16 calories, 2 grams of fiber, 2 grams of sugar, 1 gram of protein, and 81 milligrams of sodium; GL: 1.

Corn

Corn, commonly referred to as a grain food, is eaten around the world and is a staple food supply in many countries. It is also a gluten-free food. Sweet corn is a very popular variety that contains more sugar and less starch and provides approximately 123 calories per large ear. The rich fiber content of corn decreases issues of constipation and hemorrhoids and reduces the risk of colon cancer. According to the website of The World's Healthiest Foods at www.whfoods.com, corn has been found to be beneficial in managing both type 1 and type 2 diabetes by regulating the absorption and release of insulin and reducing spikes and drops in blood sugar. This naturally occurs as the result of protein and fiber in corn combining to steady the release of sugar from the digestive tract into the bloodstream.

Corn contains several phytonutrients, vitamins, minerals, and fiber; blue and purple corn varieties also have important phytonutrients. The phytochemical antioxidants in corn are known to have preventative properties in relationship to cancer and inflammation, and add a boost to the immune system; however, corn can tip the scale in terms of being acid forming in the body. Vitamin A, an active flavonoid when combined with other phytonutrients, adds extra protection against lung and oral cancers, and increases the health of the eyes and skin. Corn also contains a host of B vitamins and vitamin K working together to support normal metabolism and healthy blood clotting, and to manage blood calcium. Minerals include potassium for the regulation of heart rate and blood pressure, phosphorous, magnesium, calcium, zinc, and iron. The trace mineral selenium cooperates with vitamin E to protect the body from oxidation.

It's important to note that conventionally grown corn is a highly genetically modified food source for a variety of reasons, including increasing yield for global demand and engineering resistance to crop damage. Corn is also used to manufacture other products such as vegetable oil, high-fructose corn syrup, and so on. Anhydrous ammonia is regularly used as a base for nitrogen fertilizer in conventionally grown corn and other crops, contributing to several health and environmental safety concerns. According to organicvalley.coop, this synthetic fertilizer when it runs off and becomes a part of a water supply can create serious health issues including bladder and ovarian cancer. If you're concerned, either ask whether the corn you're purchasing is a genetically modified product utilizing synthetic fertilizers or purchase organically grown corn grown with nonchemical fertilizer from traceable organic sources whenever possible. Research is ongoing concerning the genetic engineering of food crops. One cup of yellow sweet corn contains 132 calories, 4.2 grams of fiber, 5 grams of sugar, 5 grams of protein, and 29 grams of carbohydrates; GL: 11.

Lettuce

Lettuce is a very low-calorie green food in the vegetable family, containing several vitamins, minerals, and phytonutrients, and it comes in several varieties, including romaine, crisphead (iceberg), butterhead (bibb), and leaf. The high water and fiber content in lettuce provides health to the digestive tract and removes bile salts from the body, which actually break down cholesterol as they're replenished. Romaine lettuce is a much better choice over commonly eaten iceberg lettuce, which has far lower nutritional content.

Romaine lettuce has a generous amount of vitamin K, which is essential in the proper clotting of blood and managing blood calcium levels; an abundance of vitamin A and beta-carotene, working together to provide exceptional antioxidant strength in protecting the body from lung and oral cancers and promoting growth and repair of body tissue; folate for preventing damage to blood vessels and protecting an unborn fetus; and vitamin C for its antioxidant and immune strength. Minerals in romaine lettuce include potassium for controlling blood pressure and heart rate; calcium, magnesium, and phosphorous for strengthening bones; and iron and copper for oxygen transport and red blood cell health. The minerals in romaine lettuce also help to balance the body's alkaline and acid levels, and also contain nutrients that can reduce the risk of neurodegenerative diseases by supporting healthy brain function. Antioxidants are present to protect the body from organ and tissue damage, and also contain anti-inflammatory properties that are proven to reduce and effectively control inflammation.

Be sure to wash and rinse lettuce carefully to minimize the presence of pesticides used in the conventional growing process; purchase organic whenever possible. Lettuce may also interfere with blood-thinning medications; talk with your health-care professional if this is a concern. One serving of romaine (85 grams) contains 14 calories, 2 grams of fiber, 1 gram of sugar, and 1 gram of protein; GL: 1.

Collard Greens

Collard greens are a very low-calorie, green leafy vegetable that belongs to the cruciferous family and contains no cholesterol. Collards contain an ample amount of dietary fiber, which aids in leveling blood sugar and providing health to the digestive tract by reducing constipation and the risk of colon disease. The phytochemicals in collards are great for detoxification of the body and contain a rich source of cell mutation protection against breast, ovarian, cervical, colon, and prostate cancers. Collards and other green leafy vegetables contain generous amounts of chlorophyll, which cleanses and increases the oxygen capacity of the blood and can reduce the effect of carcinogens that may be present in foods grilled at high temperatures, especially charred foods.

Collards contribute to cardiovascular health by binding and eliminating bile salts from the body, which directly impacts the lowering of cholesterol in the blood as the bile salts are replenished by the liver. Collards contain a generous amount of vitamin A and carotene, which serve as powerful antioxidants in protecting the body from oxidizing cell and tissue damage. Collards also contain B vitamins for normal nerve function, and are a generous source of folate, a B vitamin that is required for the reduction of high levels of the amino acid, homocysteine, acquired largely through meat consumption, which in high levels has been discovered to contribute to artery damage and heart disease. This green leafy vegetable also contains vitamin C for a healthy immune system and protection from cancer-causing free-radical activity, and an abundant supply of vitamin K in support of the effective management of blood calcium to protect the arteries from arterial calcification (hardening). Collards also contain a generous amount of calcium for strong bones and teeth, and other important minerals such as iron, copper, selenium, and zinc.

Be sure to wash and rinse collards to remove the pesticides used in the conventional growing process; purchase organic whenever possible. Sauté or steam collards with other flavor-adding vegetables or spices for better digestion; be careful not to overcook, thereby losing vital nutrients. Collards may interfere with blood-thinning medications and also affect individuals with thyroid and sensitive digestive tract health issues; talk to your health-care professional if these are concerns for you. One cup of chopped collards contain 11 calories, 1 gram of fiber, no sugar, and 1 gram of protein; GL: 1.

Kale

Kale is a low-calorie, phytonutrient-rich, green leafy food full of potent antioxidant properties that can place significant cancer protection around the prostate, colon, breast, bladder, and ovaries. It also aids in the detoxification of the body. Kale contains anti-inflammatory properties that cooperate with its omega 3 content to reduce the risk of painful and chronic inflammation. Kale has plenty of dietary fiber that maintains a healthy digestive tract, balances blood sugar, and can reduce constipation. Kale also binds bile salt and eliminates it from the body, subsequently reducing cholesterol during the replenishment process.

Kale contains an abundance of vitamin K, which is well documented to support bone health and normal blood clotting; a rich supply of vitamins A and C to ward off lung and oral-cavity cancers and to reduce the risk of cellular DNA damage, which is a precursor to cancer development; and a host of B vitamins. Kale is also highly regarded for its rich source of minerals, including potassium for regulating heart rate and maintaining healthy blood pressure; copper, calcium, and phosphorous for bone density; iron for transporting life-sustaining oxygen to cells and tissues; and sodium, which joins with potassium to maintain proper fluid balance in the body.

Wash and rinse kale well to remove pesticide residue; purchase organic whenever possible. Kale can be eaten as part of a mixed salad or you can sauté or steam kale with other flavor-adding vegetables or spices if digestion is an issue; be careful not to overcook, which causes a loss of vital nutrients. Kale may interfere with blood-thinning medication and also affect individuals with thyroid and sensitive digestive tract health issues; talk to your health-care professional if these are concerns. One cup of chopped kale contains 33 calories, 1 gram of fiber, no sugar, and 2 grams of protein; GL: 3.

Spinach

Spinach is a green leafy vegetable that is loaded with vitamins, minerals, and phytochemicals to discourage the growth and spread of chronic disease. Spinach is a very low-calorie green food containing an ample amount of dietary fiber that aids the regulation and balance of blood sugar and also contributes to a healthy digestive tract by protecting the tract lining and effectively eliminating toxins from the colon. Spinach is also great for weight control because of its low calorie content, and it contains specific phytonutrients that increase eye health and reduce the risk of age-related eye diseases, such as glaucoma and cataracts.

Spinach, like many green leafy foods, has a rich supply of antioxidant phytonutrients in the form of vitamins A, C, K, and a host of B vitamins, including folate, which cooperate to provide substantial health benefits, including strengthening bones through mineral retention, limiting calcium buildup in the arteries, providing antioxidant strength to boost the immune system in limiting infection, and providing significant firepower on the battlefield in the fight against the growth of free-radical activity to reduce the risk of various forms of cancer. Spinach contains an excellent supply of minerals, including iron for normal red blood cell development and aiding the transport of oxygen in the body; potassium for the regulation of blood pressure and heart rate; magnesium, manganese, and copper for bone strength; and zinc for male reproduction activity. Spinach also contains multiple anti-inflammatory properties. According to The World's Healthiest Foods at www.whfoods.com, studies have shown that spinach has demonstrated the ability to fight aggressive prostate cancer.

Wash and rinse spinach thoroughly to reduce pesticide contamination; buy organic whenever possible. Due to a high presence of oxalates (which can reduce calcium and iron absorption) and uric acid–causing purines in spinach, individuals who have kidney, gallbladder, or joint issues or are taking blood-thinning medications may want to talk to their health-care professional concerning this food. Boiling spinach is recommended to reduce the level of acids. One cup of spinach contains 7 calories, 1 gram of fiber, no sugar, and 1 gram of protein; GL: 0.

Sweet Potatoes

Sweet potatoes are a starchy root vegetable with plenty of health benefits in the form of vitamins, minerals, phytonutrients, and dietary fiber. Not to be confused with yams, sweet potatoes were originally harvested in Central and South America. According to the Library of Congress at libraryofcongress.gov, yams are native to Africa and Asia and grown primarily in Africa; starchier and drier than sweet potatoes; and less abundant in America. Sweet potatoes contain more calories than green leafy and some other vegetables; however, they contain no cholesterol and hardly any fat. Sweet potatoes are loaded with the phytonutrient beta-carotene, which converts to vitamin A in the body and is notable in its rich orange appearance. Beta-carotene may reduce the risk of breast and ovarian cancer, according to the National Institute of Health. Sweet potatoes also come in several other varieties and colors, which also contain significant antioxidant strength—particularly purple, which reportedly can reduce the risk of colorectal carcinogens, according to Dr. Joseph Mercola at www.mercola.com.

The dietary fiber in sweet potatoes contributes significantly to the health and function of the digestive tract and is well known to reduce spikes in blood sugar. Research suggests that sweet potatoes can also reduce insulin resistance in diabetics. Sweet potatoes also contain several anti-inflammatory properties as well as a host of critical vitamins, including a very generous supply of vitamin A, increasingly known to reduce the risk of lung and oral cancers as well as slowing age-related vision loss (macular degeneration); and a host of B vitamins, which are important for proper nerve function. The B vitamin folate reduces the risk of artery damage and neural tube defects in the unborn fetus, and B6 relaxes blood vessels, aiding blood flow. These jewels contain other important vitamins, such as C for immune health; K for bone strength; and E for healthy skin, hair, and immune support. Sweet potatoes also contain several important minerals, including calcium, magnesium, and phosphorous working together to increase bone density and providing aid for the proper functioning of cells, muscles, and the nervous system; manganese for metabolizing carbohydrates to maintain healthy blood-sugar levels; and a generous supply of potassium to regulate heart rate and blood pressure and maintain fluid balance in the body.

Due to the presence of oxalates in sweet potatoes, individuals with issues related to the kidneys may want to talk with their health-care professional. One medium, baked sweet potato contains 103 calories (nearly 60 less than a white potato), 3.8 grams of fiber, 7 grams of sugar, 2.29 grams of protein, 542 milligrams of potassium, and 24 grams of carbohydrates; GL: 10.

Potatoes

The potato is a starchy root vegetable, originating in South America, and today is a staple food eaten around the globe. Potatoes are rich in carbohydrates (largely complex carbs) and come in a variety of types, including russet, red skin, Yukon gold, Idaho, and several others. Potatoes are rich in vitamins, minerals, dietary fiber, phytonutrients, and starch, but contain no cholesterol and a minimal amount of fat. Starchy vegetables contain higher-energy-producing carbohydrates, which contribute to weight gain if the energy produced and stored in cells is not properly burned; the unburned energy is converted and stored as fat for later energy use.

The rich fiber content in potatoes helps prevent constipation and greatly reduces the risk of colorectal disease. The fiber content also reduces the cholesterol level in arteries and blood vessels, and at the same time works to absorb simple sugar in the stomach in support of balancing blood sugar. Potatoes are 70 percent water but contain an assortment of vitamins, including vitamins A, C, K, and B; B6 has to be singled out for its importance in aiding the development of new cells throughout the body. These vitamins also contain anti-inflammatory properties for maintaining healthy joints and tissue. Potatoes are also home to several important minerals, including a very generous amount of the electrolyte potassium for maintaining heart rate, blood pressure, and proper fluid balance; manganese to help the body utilize the antioxidants in food; calcium, magnesium, phosphorous, and copper for bone density; and iron.

To reduce sugar content, avoid refrigerating potatoes. Never purchase or eat the sprouts of potatoes or potatoes with green discoloration; they contain a toxic compound called solanine, which can create a variety of health issues including nausea and diarrhea. Frying potatoes significantly decreases their vitamin C level and contributes to blood-clogging health issues; baking, roasting, or steaming with the skin intact is preferred. If boiling, heat water to boil first to reduce cooking time and for maintaining some of the nutrients. The fiber nutrients are contained in the skin, so wash and rinse well and enjoy with the skin when possible; if necessary, peel very thinly to maintain the nutrients just below the skin. One medium, baked potato contains 161 calories, 3.8 grams of fiber, 2 grams of sugar, 4.33 grams of protein, 950 milligrams of potassium, and 37 grams of carbohydrates; GL: 17.

Green Beans

Green beans (string beans) are a pod of immature beans that contain nutritional health benefits in the form of vitamins, minerals, phytonutrients, and dietary fiber. These delicious, fresh beans are low in calories and contain no cholesterol and very little fat. They belong to the same family as pinto, black, and other beans. The dietary fiber in green beans provides a push in moving foods through the digestive tract and shields the colon from toxic substances, reducing the risk of colorectal cancer and constipation. The fiber in green beans also aids in decreasing LDL (bad) cholesterol and balancing blood-sugar levels. According to the Mateljan Foundation, research studies are showing a link between the anti-inflammatory phytonutrients in green beans and the positive role they could play in reducing type 2 diabetes.

Green beans are an excellent source of vitamins, including vitamin A, which combines with other phytonutrients, including beta-carotene, to provide cell and tissue protection and repair. Green beans contain an ample supply of vitamin C to nullify free-radical activity before it begins and provide a boost to the immune system, reducing the risk of several forms of cancer and other infectious diseases. These beans contain B vitamins and also vitamin K for strengthening bones against fractures and osteoporosis. Green beans contain several critical minerals, including iron, calcium, magnesium, phosphorous, manganese, and potassium for maintaining resilient arteries, a regular heartbeat, and healthy blood pressure.

Green beans contain significant chlorophyll, which cleanses the blood and is very helpful in battling carcinogenic agents that occur in meat that is grilled and charred at high temperatures. Frozen green beans contain more nutrients than the canned variety; it's better to eat fresh when possible. Again, don't cook the life out of them; steam or cook just enough to make them tender to enjoy. Green beans can interfere with blood-thinning medications and contain oxalic acid, which may create concerns for individuals with urinary tract issues; talk with your health-care professional as needed. One cup of green beans contain 34 calories, 4 grams of fiber, 2 grams of sugar, and 2 grams of protein; GL: 3.

Green Peas

Green peas contain starch and are part of the legume (bean) family. The peas are removed from their pods just prior to reaching full maturity when they are sweet and tender; they're fairly low in calories and contain no cholesterol. Peas are rich in dietary fiber and protein, which combine to slow digestion of food into usable sugar and are helpful in maintaining a healthy digestive system and blood-sugar balance. Omega 3 fatty acids combine with the rich anti-inflammatory phytonutrients to reduce the risk and harsh effects of inflammation. These phytonutrients have also been shown to reduce incidents of stomach cancer.

These green warriors are an excellent source of vitamins, minerals, and phytonutrients. Peas contain an ample supply of vitamin A, and when combined with their carotenoid properties, become fierce fighters in battling lung and oral cancers and degenerative eye disease. Vitamin B in peas provides energy metabolism and excellent nervous system protection. The phytonutrients in vitamin C are amazing in shielding the body from cancer-causing free-radical invasion, destroying their growth and development to reduce the risk of cellular DNA damage. Vitamin K balances blood calcium and strengthens bones. Green peas contain several minerals, including an ample supply of copper, manganese, potassium, and zinc.

Green peas contain purines that contribute to the development of uric acid in the body. Individuals with issues associated with the kidneys or joint inflammation should consult with their health-care professional concerning this food. One cup of green peas contain 117 calories, 7 grams of fiber, 8 grams of sugar, and 8 grams of protein; GL: 8.

Asparagus

Asparagus is a green vegetable (available in other varietal colors) belonging to the lily family with onions and garlic. It's low in calories and contains no fat, but does contain a wide variety of vitamins, minerals, phytonutrients, and dietary fiber. The fiber content in asparagus serves to protect the colon from toxic materials and joins with the vegetable's protein content to slow the digestion of food into usable sugar, resulting in better regulation of blood-sugar levels. According to the *British Journal of Nutrition*, asparagus improves insulin secretion, which aids in controlling blood-sugar levels as well. Asparagus also decreases LDL (bad) cholesterol and contains an amino acid that acts as a diuretic in expelling water, excess salt, and toxins from the body.

This spear-shaped vegetable has a rich amount of vitamin A; B vitamins, including folate; a modest amount of vitamin C; and a rich supply of vitamin K for aiding in the mineralization of bones, regulating blood calcium to prevent arterial calcification, and maintaining proper blood clotting to prevent bleeding issues. Asparagus also contains important minerals, including iron, copper, potassium, and the bone doctors calcium, phosphorous, and magnesium to maintain bone density and strength. Asparagus also has sizable antioxidant strength for preventing oxidation damage to healthy cells and tissues, thereby reducing the risk of cancer activity; asparagus also has an excellent anti-inflammatory capacity.

Wash and rinse asparagus well before cooking; buy organic when possible. To protect the extensive nutrients, cook just enough to make tender. Grilling or sautéing are the preferred cooking methods; it can also be consumed raw in other dishes. Asparagus may produce a light odor in the urine due to its sulfur content. Asparagus contains purines, which produce uric acid; individuals with kidney or joint issues should consult with their health-care professional concerning this food. Half a cup of cooked asparagus contains 20 calories, 1.8 grams of fiber, 1 gram of sugar, and 2.16 grams of protein; GL: 2.

Zucchini

Zucchini, also considered a fruit, is a member of the summer squash family and originated in Central America and Mexico. Zucchini is varietal, and a few of those varieties are dark green, golden, and courgette. Other summer squash varieties include yellow crookneck and straight neck; winter squashes include the popular acorn and butternut varieties. Zucchini is low in calories and contains hardly any fat and no cholesterol. Zucchini is an excellent source of dietary fiber, which aids in moving food through the complete digestive tract, supporting the health of the colon and reducing the risk of constipation and colorectal disease. Zucchini also has generous water content at 95 percent and combines with fiber to satisfy the appetite, which can aid weight reduction and hydration. According to the website Organic Facts at www.organicfacts.net, zucchini can decrease enlarged prostate symptoms in men.

Zucchini contains important vitamins, minerals, and phytonutrients that aid in providing substantial health benefits. The golden zucchini has an abundant supply of the phytonutrient carotene, which attacks and limits free-radical development, adds nutrients for eye health, and partners with the omega 3 fatty acid content to reduce the risk of inflammatory diseases such as arthritis and asthma. Zucchini contains B vitamins, vitamin C is in ample supply, and vitamins A and K are also present in this amazing food. The mineral potassium in zucchini regulates heart rate and blood pressure and maintains fluid balance. Zucchini also contains a combination of calcium, magnesium, phosphorous, and manganese to accomplish a variety of tasks, including enabling healthy bone structure.

Wash and rinse zucchini well before consuming and avoid peeling because of the rich fiber content of the skin. Purchase organic when possible. Zucchini can be eaten raw or prepared in a variety of ways, including steamed, baked, or combined with other veggies in stews or casseroles. Consuming zucchini and summer squash can produce oxalic acid; individuals with kidney issues may want to talk to their healthcare professional concerning this food. One medium zucchini contains 33 calories, 2 grams of fiber, 4.9 grams of sugar, and 2.4 grams of protein; GL: 0.

Beets

Beets are a root vegetable, a beautiful deep red in color, low in calories, and contain no cholesterol and a very small amount of fat. Beets contain an ample amount of dietary fiber, which plays a major role in maintaining a healthy digestive tract, including the health of the colon; the fiber also aids in lowering LDL (bad) cholesterol and triglycerides in the blood. Beets also contain sufficient carbohydrates to produce energy for an active lifestyle and are a natural blood cleanser, providing vital support to the liver. Beets also supply nitric oxide to the blood, which relaxes blood vessels, improving blood flow.

Beets contain a variety of vitamins, including vitamin A; B vitamins; vitamin C, with its immense power in sustaining a healthy immune system; and smaller amounts of vitamins E and K. Several important minerals are present in beets, including potassium, iron, copper, manganese, magnesium for bone mineralization, and zinc for wound healing and male reproduction. Beet greens are an edible part of the plant and also contain several vitamins and minerals. Beets also contain a phytonutrient that reduces the amino acid, homocysteine, in the blood supply, greatly reducing the risk of blood-vessel damage. According to www.organicfacts.net, beets can counteract cancerous cell growth in the prevention of cancers of the lung, colon, and skin. Beets also stand guard against the cancerous compounds caused by nitrate preservatives placed in meat.

Beets have very high sugar content but a slow release; sugar beets are used for making refined white sugar. Beets contain oxalates; persons with issues related to the kidneys should talk with their health-care professional concerning this food. One cup of beets contains 58 calories, 4 grams of fiber, 9 grams of sugar, and 2 grams of protein; GL: 5.

Onions

> *"We remember the fish we ate in Egypt at no cost—also the cucumbers, melons, leeks, onions, and garlic."*
> —NUMBERS 11:5 (NIV)

Onion is a pungent bulb vegetable, belonging to the allium family that can literally bring you to tears due to the release of sulfur compounds when sliced. The onion is very low in calories and fat, contains no cholesterol, and comes in several varieties, including red (great for salads), yellow (great for cooking), white, and bunching (green onions). Onions contain fiber to balance blood sugar and provide support to maintain the healthy bacteria in the colon, which contributes to the overall health of the digestive system.

Onions are rich in vitamins, minerals, and phytonutrients that have been used for health and healing for thousands of years. When sliced, onion's potent phytonutrient allicin (which contains sulfur compounds) has been shown to lower the risk of various cancers, including stomach and colon cancers; it also provides cures in different areas of the body, including the mouth and digestive tract, due to its antiviral and antibacterial properties. Phytonutrient compounds in onions provide nitric oxide to the blood supply, which relaxes blood vessels and creates better blood flow, and are also beneficial in reducing LDL (bad) cholesterol, reducing the risk of coronary disease and stroke. Phytonutrients in onions have the capacity to lower blood-sugar levels and reduce inflammation in the body, greatly reducing the discomfort and inflammatory pain of arthritis and gout.

Onions contain a variety of minerals, including manganese, phosphorous, magnesium, potassium, iron, calcium, copper, zinc, and the trace mineral chromium, which supports insulin in the proper absorption of glucose into the cells for energy, thereby promoting healthy blood-sugar levels. Vitamins are also in ample supply in onions, including a host of B vitamins. Vitamin C is also in generous supply for building and sustaining a robust immune system in its battle to defeat the growth of cancerous free radicals and facilitating a simultaneous fight to reduce infection in the body.

Always use a sharp knife when slicing and chopping onions; you don't want to cry and chop in front of your friends any longer than necessary. Don't overpeel an onion after removing the outer wrap; many of the nutrients are contained in the outer layers. One medium onion contains 44 calories, 2 grams of fiber, 5 grams of sugar, and 1 gram of protein; GL: 4.

Garlic

Mentioned in the scriptures (Numbers 11:5), garlic is a bulb plant that originated in Central Asia and belongs to the allium family along with its onion cousin. Garlic contains several vitamins, minerals, and phytonutrients that provide substantial health benefits. Similar to onions, garlic contains the phytonutrient allicin, which is created when the garlic bulb is cut or crushed. Garlic's pungent aroma comes from the sulfur contained in allicin. Studies have shown allicin to be effective in reducing the risk of several cancers, including stomach and colon cancer. Allicin is an effective antiviral and antibacterial agent, particularly in the mouth and stomach areas. Phytonutrients in garlic are well known to produce nitrous oxide, which provides flexibility in blood vessels and reduces blood pressure, and also significantly reduces LDL (bad) cholesterol in the blood; combined, these health attributes reduce the risk of coronary artery disease and stroke.

Garlic contains a wide and rich source of minerals, including potassium, magnesium, phosphorous, calcium, zinc, manganese for calcium absorption and proper thyroid function, iron for transporting oxygen to cells and tissues throughout the body, and selenium for antioxidant support. Garlic also contains an ample supply of vitamin C for immune health and B vitamins, including vitamin B6, which aids the development of new red blood cells and contributes to healthy blood vessels.

There is nothing like the pungent, aromatic smell and taste of garlic in many of our favorite dishes. Garlic is said to have unpleasant odors when eaten, quite the contrary, garlic on the breath signifies its active ingredients at work providing its several health benefits. Garlic may interfere with blood-thinning medications; talk to your health-care professional if this is a concern. One clove of garlic (the small section within the bulb) contains four calories, 0 fiber, 0 sugars, and 0 proteins; GL: 0.

Bell Peppers

Bell pepper is native to Central America and is a member of the nightshade family of vegetables, which includes its hot relatives cayenne, jalapeño, and habaneras. Bell pepper contains very little fat and no cholesterol, and contains important dietary fiber, which supports healthy digestion and cholesterol levels. Based on their variety, bell peppers become bright, beautiful colors such as red, yellow, and orange as they mature. Red bell peppers contain excellent levels of antioxidants and anti-inflammatory phytochemicals, including beta-carotene, which reduces the risk of chronic cell diseases, and lycopene, which provides the rich red color and acts as a partner in reducing cancer-causing cell damage. Yellow and orange peppers are rich in carotenoids as well.

Bell peppers, particularly red, contain a very generous supply of vitamin C, which is heralded as one of the most important antioxidants in the prevention of cell destruction, binding free-radical development before it can begin its evil and cancerous devastation. Bell peppers are an excellent source of vitamin A, B vitamins, vitamin E, and vitamin K for its superior ability to reduce the risk of artery calcification. Critical minerals include manganese for helping the body to properly utilize antioxidants and support calcium absorption; potassium for regulating a healthy heartbeat and blood pressure; iron for transporting oxygen throughout the body; magnesium, phosphorous and calcium for strengthening bones; copper for improved iron absorption and utilization; and zinc.

Wash and rinse bell peppers to avoid the harmful effects of pesticides used during the conventional growing process; purchase organic whenever possible. Eat raw or cook lightly to maintain vital nutrients, especially vitamin C. Individuals with joint issues may want to talk with their health-care professional concerning the consumption of vegetables in the nightshade family. One medium bell pepper contains 24 calories, 2 grams of fiber, 3 grams of sugar, and 1 gram of protein; GL: 2.

Okra

Okra, also known as lady's finger, originated in Africa and is very low in calories and contains very little fat and no cholesterol. Okra has a generous supply of dietary fiber to support the movement of food through the entire digestive tract, reducing the risk of colorectal disease and chronic constipation. The fiber in okra is also helpful in lowering bad cholesterol and regulating blood sugar.

Okra contains an ample amount of vitamin A and beta-carotene to lower the risk of lung and oral cancers and to reduce aged-related eye diseases, such as cataracts. Okra is a great resource for B vitamins and vitamin C, and contains an ample supply of vitamin K for supporting bone mineralization in reducing the risk of osteoporosis. Okra also contains a wide variety of minerals, including a rich amount of manganese for healthy thyroid function and proper utilization of antioxidants; potassium for healthy blood pressure; magnesium, phosphorous, and calcium for rigid and healthy bones; copper for iron absorption; and zinc for healing wounds.

Buy okra fresh and eat as fresh as possible to absorb the vital nutrients. Okra is used often in gumbo dishes. Wash and rinse thoroughly to eliminate pesticide residue; buy organic if available. Select the smaller healthy plants for their tender quality. Okra contains oxalates; individuals with kidney or gallbladder issues may want to talk to their health-care professional concerning this food. Half a cup of cooked okra contains 18 calories, 2 grams of fiber, 2 grams of sugar, and 1.5 grams of protein; GL: 2.

Summary
Many of the aforementioned vegetables can be eaten raw or cooked—your choice. However, some of the vegetables, such as potatoes, sweet potatoes, corn, dark green leafy vegetables, and others, are better cooked for digestibility. However, if you're cooking your vegetables, steam or sauté at low temperature just long enough to make them tender in order to retain as many of the nutrients as possible; you don't want to consume a plate of completely devitalized food.

A few vegetables retain much of their nutrient value after light steaming, such as asparagus, broccoli, carrots, green beans, and onions. Vegetables such as spinach lose more than half of their vitamin C during cooking. The nutrients in tomatoes, particularly their lycopene content, are better absorbed following cooking, which is why men challenged with prostate issues are encouraged to eat tomato sauces in addition to raw tomatoes. Either way, prepare vegetables in a way that you're most likely to eat and properly digest them. If you have concerns, consult with your health-care professional concerning the issue of consuming raw or cooked vegetables.

Food for Thought

- For highest nutrition, eat fresh vegetables and organic if available, and purchase fresh from trusted local farm sources or stores that utilize local farm sources when possible.
- Don't cook the life out of your vegetables; steam or sauté until tender but not mushy.
- Vegetable juice can be consumed in place of whole vegetables; talk to your health-care provider to determine if this aligns with your health status and goals.
- Men should eat fresh and cooked tomatoes for prostate health; tomatoes are also an excellent source of potassium.
- Vegetables are a building food; five half-cup servings daily are recommended.
- Eat a variety of vegetables, including nutrient-rich green leafy vegetables for healthy blood, a healthy heart, and antioxidant cell protection from free-radical activity.
- Cruciferous vegetables like broccoli, cabbage, and brussels sprouts are effective in shielding the body from several cancers, including cancers of the breast, colon, prostate, pancreas, and

bladder. According to the National Cancer Institute, cruciferous vegetables can inhibit tumor blood vessel formation and tumor cell migration (restricting tumor travel). These vegetables can also breakdown estrogen for elimination in the urine; further reducing the risk of estrogen related cancers such as cancers of the breast and prostate.

- Carrots and sweet potatoes contain generous amounts of the cancer-fighting "angel" beta-carotene; carrots juice well with other fruits and vegetables.
- Carrots are well known for being a cleansing agent for the liver and for removing harmful metals, such as aluminum, from the fatty tissue in the body, which can reduce the risk of neurodegenerative disorders such as Alzheimer's disease.
- Never purchase or eat the sprouts of potatoes or potatoes with green discoloration; they contain a toxic compound called solanine, which contributes to multiple health issues.
- Spinach has demonstrated the ability to fight aggressive prostate cancer; however, vegetables such as spinach that contain high levels of oxalates and purines can possibly contribute to complications in the urinary tract; talk to your health-care professional as necessary.
- Tomatoes and celery expel toxins and uric acid from the body, reducing incidents of urinary tract infections.
- Onions contain the trace mineral chromium, which supports insulin in the proper absorption of glucose into the cells for energy, thereby promoting healthy blood-sugar levels; fiber contributes to healthy bacteria in the colon.
- The lignan phytonutrients contained in cucumbers have the ability to reduce the risk of estrogen-related cancers, such as cancers of the breast, ovaries, uterus, and prostate.
- Zucchini is known to aid in decreasing enlarged prostate symptoms in men.

Close

This chapter concludes information concerning the two most important food groups known to humankind: fruits and vegetables. The powerful health-sustaining properties in these two food groups are undeniable. I hope you've learned something new and have been inspired by the information in this chapter and the preceding one to take the necessary steps to include more fresh fruits and vegetables in your diet. It's an important step when you consider that approximately 13.1 percent of the American adult population meets the recommended standard for fruit and 8.9 percent for vegetable consumption, according to the Center for Disease Control and Prevention (CDC) as reported in *Medical News Today*.

You will be amazed at what regular consumption within these two food groups will do for your health and the health of your family. Look them all over and select and enjoy those that are right for you; talk to your health-care professional as appropriate. It's also important to note that you should purchase fresh produce as often as possible from trusted local farms or from stores that utilize local sources; these fruits and vegetables will be fresher and on the shelf faster, and will contain more vitamins, minerals, and phytonutrients than produce trucked across the country. Finally, exercise care in consuming large quantities of vegetable and fruit combinations in smoothies and other mixtures. The body is equipped to handle food nutrients in required human levels; don't go overboard. Talk to your health-care provider if you're consuming large quantities of food for specific health reasons.

Recall the words of God our Father in Genesis 1:29 concerning fruit, and the words of Daniel 1:11–15 concerning the tremendous attributes of vegetables as you're making your decision related to increasing your fresh fruit and vegetable intake. As a sensible and intelligent individual, I think you understand the reason your path has placed you in contact with this information. Take charge of providing higher nutrition for you and your family!

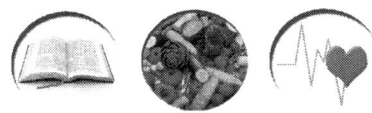

CHAPTER 3

NUTS AND SEEDS

*"Then their father Israel said to them, 'If it must be,
then do this: Put some of the best product of the
land in your bags and take them down to the man as
a gift—a little balm and a little honey, some spices
and myrrh, some pistachios nuts and almonds.'"*
—GENESIS 43:11 (NIV)

It's interesting that a man's simple request to Israel's sons (unbeknown to them, the man was actually their brother Joseph) to return to him with their youngest brother Benjamin in order to purchase more food for their family would cause their father Israel to pack their most precious gifts for the man, including a precious commodity among their possessions: pistachios and almonds. A little amazing when thousands of years later you can easily bridge the historic and precious value of these two items to their nutritious value today.

Today, nuts are a large part of the American diet and should be eaten as part of an overall balanced diet. Nuts contain ample amounts of heart-healthy, monounsaturated fatty acids, which can be burned quickly for energy; some contain the anti-inflammatory support source omega 3 fatty acid. These fatty acids have demonstrated their ability to reduce LDL (bad) cholesterol and increase HDL (good) cholesterol to support a healthy heart and cardiovascular system. Nuts and seeds contain an ample supply of various phytonutrients to protect the body from free-radical cell damage and chronic inflammatory health issues. Nuts and seeds are also a gluten-free food, and contain protein to strengthen muscle and provide support for immune health. Carbohydrates in nuts supply the body with energy.

Nuts are a great source of B vitamins and the antioxidant vitamin E, which stops plaque buildup in the arteries and reduces the risk of free-radical activity in the body. Nuts and seeds are extremely rich in minerals for supporting a healthy bone structure, muscle and nervous system function, proper cell function, oxygen transport, and wound healing. These minerals also play a role in manufacturing protein, generating energy, controlling blood pressure and heart rate, and several other important functions and activities. Essential minerals on the scene include copper, magnesium, phosphorous, manganese, iron, potassium, and more. Nuts are a good source of fiber for balancing blood sugar, aiding the control of diabetes, and supporting a healthy digestive and colon tract.

There's a lot of discussion concerning the health benefits of raw nuts versus roasted nuts. Here are a few important things for you to know. If you're consuming roasted nuts, it's important to purchase dry roasted nuts versus nuts that contain oil; be sure no oil is listed on the package. According to Dr. Daniel Heller, naturopathic physician, nuts that contain oil are likely fried rather than roasted, creating an unhealthy fried food—an important distinction when making healthy food choices. Roasting has other risks according to the online site at healthyeating.sfgate.com and other information sites. The high-heat roasting process creates carcinogenic acrylamides; tread carefully! Needless to say, be careful to eat fewer salted nuts to maintain a healthy blood pressure.

You should also be aware that raw nuts are healthier when they have been properly soaked and dried to remove naturally occurring phytic acid; a substance that can interrupt your body's ability to absorb important minerals, including iron, calcium, magnesium, and zinc (see Phytic Acid under Things You Should Know). If the soaking process is too cumbersome and you're interested in purchasing or discovering additional information concerning raw nuts that have undergone this preparation, you can visit the website of Wilderness Family Naturals at www.wildernessfamilynaturals.com; you can visit other sites as well.

Although they contain multiple health benefits, nuts are known to be acid forming in addition to containing ample fat and calories, so enjoy nuts sparingly. Questions concerning the consumption of this food should be directed to your health-care professional. The nut and seed nutrient profile is included at the end of each description, including the glycemic load (GL), which measures the amount of carbohydrate in food converting to sugar and its effect on blood sugar.

Glycemic Load: Low = 10 or less; Medium = 11–19; High = 20 and above

Almonds

Almonds are the seed of the fruit of the almond tree; they're grown in California and other places around the world and contain an ample supply of vitamins, minerals, and phytonutrients. Almonds contain the proper balance of monounsaturated fatty acids that contribute to lowering cholesterol, and according to the George Mateljan Foundation, almonds have the ability to increase antioxidants and lower blood-sugar and insulin levels.

Almonds contain a rich supply of the antioxidant vitamin E, which helps protect cells from free-radical damage and contributes to healthy skin and hair. Almonds are also a source of B vitamins for energy metabolism, cell development, healthy muscle and nerve function, and maintaining healthy arteries. Almonds contain a rich supply of important minerals, such as potassium for heart health; iron for oxygen transport and red blood cell formation; calcium for bone strength; magnesium for healthy blood flow; zinc for healing wounds; and other important minerals, including manganese, for metabolizing carbohydrates and healthy thyroid function.

Almonds do contain oxalates, which may affect individuals with kidney or gallbladder issues; talk to your health-care professional if this is a concern for you. Individuals with allergies to tree nuts may also want to talk to their health-care professional concerning this food. One ounce of almonds (23 nuts) contains 162 calories, 14 grams total fat, no cholesterol, 6 grams of protein, 3 grams of fiber, and 1 gram of sugar; GL: 0.

Walnuts

Walnuts are a varietal part of the tree nut family, including English, black, and white (butternut). Walnuts contain healthy omega 3 fatty acids and monounsaturated fatty acids, which burn quickly in providing energy and stimulating brain activity, and also play an important role in lowering cholesterol and blood pressure, contributing to overall heart health. The fatty acids can reduce inflammation in the body and reduce the risk of colon, breast, and prostate cancers, especially when combined with the rich phytonutrients in walnuts. Walnuts have a generous supply of fiber, which supports a healthy digestive tract. Walnuts support the reproductive health of men and aid in the control of diabetes by impacting insulin levels.

Walnuts are rich in vitamin E, which provides support for a healthy immune system and protection from free-radical damage. They are also a rich source of B vitamins, including folate, which protects against neural tube defects during pregnancy and maintains healthy arteries. Walnuts are a very rich source of minerals, especially copper for iron absorption and utilization; manganese for aiding calcium absorption; phosphorous for healthy cell function and bone structure; magnesium for proper muscle and nerve function; zinc for wound healing; and potassium for aiding healthy blood pressure and heart rate, as well as calcium, iron, and selenium.

Individuals with allergies to tree nuts may want to talk to their health-care professional concerning this food. An ounce of walnuts (14 halves) contains 185 calories, 18 grams total fat, no cholesterol, 4 grams of protein, 2 grams of fiber, and 1 gram of sugar; GL: 0.

Pecans

Pecans belong to the tree nut (hickory) family and are an excellent source of antioxidants, minerals, and vitamins. Pecans are native to the United States and second in popularity behind peanuts. Pecans contain a generous supply of healthy monounsaturated fatty acids, which help to reduce blood cholesterol and prevent artery disease and stroke. The pecan is the most antioxidant-rich tree nut, and its combination of phytonutrients, including vitamin E and beta-carotene, teams up to battle free-radical oxidation, which significantly reduce the risk of cancer and other chronic diseases. Pecans are a rich source of fiber, which aids in maintaining a healthy digestive tract.

Pecans are also a rich source of B vitamins for normal growth and development, protein metabolism, proper nervous system function, red blood cell production, healthy arteries, and the normal function of muscles, including the heart muscle. Pecans contain a generous supply of minerals, especially manganese and copper for healthy bone structure and red blood cell formation; zinc for maintaining healthy immune function and healthy male reproduction; phosphorous for overall healthy cell function; and potassium for regulating blood pressure and heart rate; as well as iron, calcium, selenium, and magnesium.

Persons with allergies to tree nuts may want to talk to their healthcare professional concerning this food. One ounce of pecans (19 halves) contains 195 calories, 20 grams total fat, no cholesterol, 3 grams of protein, 3 grams of fiber, and 1 gram of sugar; GL: 0.

Pistachios

Pistachios are a tree nut native to Asia. They contain essential vitamins, minerals, and phytonutrients and are a generous source of monounsaturated fatty acids, which contribute heavily to the reduction of cholesterol in the blood, actually increasing HDL (good) cholesterol.

Pistachios contain a rich supply of phytochemicals in the form of vitamin E and carotenoids that bind free-radical development, simultaneously increasing immune health and lowering the risk of chronic disease, including cancer. Pistachios are a rich source of protein and are the richest source of potassium of all the nuts, regulating blood pressure and heart rate. Pistachios are rich in B vitamins, especially thiamin for proper nervous system and heart function, and vitamin B6 for red blood cell development and healthy arteries. Vitamins A and C are also present in ample supply. Like several nuts, pistachios contain a very generous amount of the mineral copper, which plays an active role in the development of red blood cells; a generous supply of manganese, phosphorous, iron, magnesium, calcium, and zinc are also present.

According to Organic Facts at www.organicfacts.net, pistachios are known to increase sexual vitality in men. Individuals with tree nut allergies should talk with their health-care professional concerning this food. One ounce of pistachios (47 nuts) contains 158 calories, 13 grams total fat, no cholesterol, 6 grams of protein, 3 grams of fiber, 292 milligrams of potassium, and 2 grams of sugar; GL: 1.

Cashews

Cashews are tree nuts native to Brazil and are picked from the cashew fruit, also known as the cashew apple. Cashews are an excellent source of monounsaturated fatty acids, which are great for the heart and cardiovascular system due to their ability to lower LDL (bad) cholesterol and increase HDL (good) cholesterol. Cashews can reduce triglyceride levels, which helps in the control of diabetes. Raw cashews are not truly raw due to being heated to remove them from their toxic shell, which is why cashews are only available outside of the shell.

Cashews contain very rich supplies of the minerals copper, for supporting healthy bones and iron absorption, and phosphorous, for cell function. Iron, potassium, calcium, selenium, and zinc are also present for delivering their specific health benefits. Cashews also contain a rich supply of vitamin E, which joins with the mineral selenium to provide antioxidant protection in the fight against free-radical development. A host of B vitamins are present, including vitamin B6 for red blood cell development and artery protection, thiamin (B1) for nerve and muscle function, pantothenic acid (B5) for energy metabolism and normal growth and development, and vitamin K for proper blood clotting and balancing blood calcium levels in reducing calcification of the arteries.

Individuals with tree nut allergies may need to consult their health-care professional concerning this food. Cashews also contain oxalates; individuals with kidney or gallstone issues may also need to consult with their health-care provider concerning this food. One ounce of raw cashews contains 155 calories, 12 grams total fat, no cholesterol, 5 grams of protein; 1 gram of fiber, and 2 grams of sugar; GL: 3.

Macadamia Nuts

Macadamia nuts are native to Australia and contain one of the higher calorie contents among nuts. Macadamia nuts contain a generous supply of monounsaturated fatty acids (rivaling those found in olive oil), which is great for lowering LDL (bad) cholesterol in the blood and contributing to a reduced risk of coronary artery disease. The fiber in macadamia nuts can reduce hunger, slow digestion in regulating blood sugar, and contribute to a healthy digestive tract, reducing the risk of colorectal disease and constipation. The protein in macadamia and other nuts helps to grow and repair muscle and support a healthy immune system.

Macadamia nuts are a rich source of B vitamins, particularly thiamin (B1) for proper nerve function, maintaining healthy heart muscle, and energy metabolism. Other B vitamins provided include B6 for red blood cell development, pantothenic acid (B5) for normal growth and development, and niacin (B3) for healthy skin. Macadamia nuts contain small amounts of the antioxidant vitamins C and E for maintaining a healthy immune system and reducing the risk of infection and chronic disease. The mineral manganese is in very rich supply for helping the body to properly utilize antioxidants, supporting bone strength, and aiding in the absorption of calcium and proper function of the thyroid. These nuts contain an ample supply of potassium in addition to magnesium, iron, copper, phosphorous, calcium, and zinc.

Individuals with nut allergies may want to talk with their health-care professional concerning this food. One ounce of macadamia nuts (11 nuts) contains 201 calories, 21 grams total fat, no cholesterol, 2 grams of protein, 2 grams of fiber, and 1 gram of sugar; GL: 0.

Brazil Nuts

Brazil nuts are a tree nut grown in several areas of the Amazon forest and contain a healthy supply of monounsaturated fatty acids, which support a healthy cardiovascular system due to their ability to decrease LDL (bad) cholesterol and increase HDL (good cholesterol, thereby protecting the body from artery disease. The brazil nut contains a sizable amount of complete protein, which is used for building and repairing tissue for normal growth and development and supporting the health of the immune system.

Brazil nuts contain a rich supply of vitamin E, which serves as an oxidant in protecting the body's tissues and cells from free-radical damage, while providing support for healthy hair and skin and a healthy immune system. Brazil nuts are a good source for B vitamins and the tremendous health benefits they provide. They're especially rich in thiamin (B1) for converting carbohydrates into energy and maintaining proper function of the heart, muscles, and nervous system. Brazil nuts also contain important minerals and are especially rich in copper, phosphorous, and magnesium, which contribute to sturdy and healthy bone structure, healthy cell function, absorption of iron, protein building, respiratory health, and more. An ample amount of potassium is available to ensure the regulation of blood pressure and heart rate.

Brazil nuts do contain a very high level of the antioxidant support mineral selenium, which, according to several sources, can be toxic if eaten in excess of the daily upper intake level of 400 mcg, equivalent to five brazil nuts. Talk to your health-care provider if you have any concerns related to this precaution or if you have tree nut allergies. One ounce of brazil nuts (approximately 6 to 7 nuts) contains 184 calories, 19 grams total fat, no cholesterol, 4 grams of protein, 2 grams of fiber, and 1 gram of sugar; GL: 0.

Pumpkin Seeds

Pumpkins are native to Mexico and are part of the squash family; their seeds are commonly known as pumpkin seeds or pepitas. The seeds contain fiber for maintaining digestive health and have an ample supply of healthy monounsaturated fatty acids that contribute significantly to heart health by lowering cholesterol, reducing the risk of coronary artery disease. The seeds also contain an ample amount of protein that works to grow and repair body tissue and provide support for a healthy immune system. According to mercola.com, pumpkin seeds provide a variety of health benefits, including supporting prostate health, specifically in the treatment of an enlarged prostate. The seeds also battle parasites in the intestinal tract, and their oil can be used in controlling menopausal conditions in postmenopausal women.

Pumpkin seeds are a generous source of specific amino acids and B vitamins. They're a generous source of niacin (B3), which actually aids in the reduction of LDL (bad) cholesterol and promotes healthy skin, and the B vitamin folate, which contributes to healthy blood vessels and reduces the risk of neural tube defects during pregnancy. A rich level of vitamin E is present, which acts to boost the immune system; vitamin C is also available in a small supply. Minerals are especially rich in pumpkin seeds, particularly manganese and phosphorous, which cooperate to ensure the body utilizes antioxidants effectively and properly absorbs calcium. They also ensure proper cell function and support healthy bone structure. Copper, iron, magnesium, selenium, calcium, and zinc are also present.

Pumpkin seeds are alkaline in the body. Eat pumpkin seeds raw to receive the highest level of nutrients (see Phytic Acid under Things You Should Know). If roasting, cook for fifteen to twenty minutes in the oven at a temperature of about 170 degrees Fahrenheit. Individuals with nut or seed allergies should talk to their health-care professional concerning this food. One ounce of pumpkin seeds contains 125 calories, 15 grams total carbohydrates, 5 grams total fat, no cholesterol, 5 grams of protein, 0 grams of fiber, and 0 grams of sugar; GL: 10.

Sunflower Seeds

Sunflower seeds are native to the United States. They are especially rich in polyunsaturated fatty acids and also contain a good source of monounsaturated fatty acid, which has the ability to lower LDL (bad) cholesterol and increase HDL (good) cholesterol in the blood, reducing the risk of artery damage and supporting heart health. Sunflower seeds have a generous supply of complete protein for supporting immune health and growing and repairing tissue, which contributes to normal growth and development. The seeds also contain the necessary fiber to aid the health of the digestive tract and provide support for balancing blood sugar. The phytonutrient carotene is present in sunflower seeds to reduce the risk and development of free radicals before they can cause cellular DNA damage.

Sunflower seeds contain an excellent supply of B vitamins, especially thiamin (B1) for the proper function of the heart, muscles, and nervous system, and a rich supply of vitamin B6 for blood-vessel protection; a rich supply of folate is also available. Vitamin E is in generous supply in the seeds to boost the immune system and to place the proper prevention around cellular and tissue oxidation. Vitamins A and C are in moderate supply to reduce the risk of lung and oral-cavity cancers and reduce the risk of infection. Minerals are also in ample supply, particularly copper for its ability to increase the absorption and utilization of iron. Phosphorous, magnesium, manganese, potassium, calcium, iron, and zinc are also present to provide their healthy contributions.

Individuals with nut or seed allergies should talk to their health-care professional concerning this food. One ounce of sunflower seeds contains 164 calories, 14 grams total fat, no cholesterol, 6 grams of protein, 2 grams of fiber, and 1 gram of sugar; GL: 0.

Sesame Seeds

Sesame seeds are native to Africa and India. They contain a generous amount of omega 6 fatty acids and an ample supply of monounsaturated fatty acids for support of the cardiovascular system, contributing to the decrease of LDL (bad) cholesterol and increasing HDL (good) cholesterol in the blood, which significantly reduces the risk of coronary artery disease and stroke. The seeds contain a generous amount of complete protein for building and repairing tissue and supporting the health of the immune system. Sesame seeds also contain a generous amount of fiber that acts to support the health of the digestive system, including the colon tract, and regulates blood sugar in supporting the control of diabetes. The seeds contain several phytochemicals that lend vital support in arresting free-radical activity, limiting their attack on healthy cells.

Like many seeds and nuts, sesame seeds contain a rich supply of B vitamins, including B6 for cell development and healthy blood vessels; thiamin (B1) for proper heart, muscle, and nervous system function;

niacin (B3) for lowering LDL (bad) cholesterol; folate (a B vitamin) for reducing the risk of neural tube defects during pregnancy; and riboflavin (B2) to protect against cataracts and facilitate carbohydrate energy conversion and red blood cell formation. Vitamin E is also available for boosting the immune system and contributing to healthy skin and hair. Sesame seeds contain a very generous supply of copper, which effectively aids in the absorption of iron, forms new red blood cells, and provides arthritic inflammation relief. Iron is in generous supply for transporting oxygen to tissue and cells. Phosphorous, magnesium, calcium, potassium, manganese, selenium, and zinc are also present.

Sesame seeds are used to make the tahini paste used in hummus. Individuals with nut or seed allergies should talk to their health-care professional concerning this food. One ounce of sesame seeds contains 158 calories, 13 grams total fat, no cholesterol, 5 grams of protein, 4 grams of fiber, and 0 grams of sugar; GL: 0.

Food for Thought:

- Although they contain healthy fat, nuts are acidic and contain a fairly high amount of fat; eat sparingly.
- Improved mineral and nutritional absorption occurs following proper soaking and drying of raw nuts and seeds.
- If eating roasted nuts, eat dry roasted nuts opposed to nuts cooked in oil; be careful not to overconsume due to carcinogenic concerns associated with roasted nuts.
- For healthy blood pressure and cardiovascular health, eat unsalted nuts.
- Brazil nuts, sunflower seeds, and sesame seeds contain complete protein; observe precautions concerning brazil nuts' selenium content.

- Pistachios are a great source of potassium and their monoun-saturated fatty acids increases HDL (good cholesterol).
- The pecan is the most antioxidant-rich tree nut, and its combination of phytonutrients teams up to battle free-radical oxidation, which significantly reduces the risk of cancer and other chronic diseases.
- Walnuts contain healthy omega 3 fatty acids and monounsaturated fatty acids, which burn quickly to provide energy and stimulate brain activity. Walnuts also play an important role in lowering cholesterol and blood pressure, contributing to overall heart health.
- Pumpkin seeds support prostate health, provides relief for menopausal conditions, and can battle parasites in the intestinal tract.
- Nuts and seeds are gluten-free foods, and contain protein for strengthening muscles and supporting immune health.

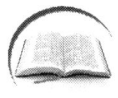 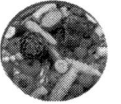 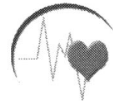

BEANS

*"When David came to Mahanaim, Shobi son of Nahash
from Rabbah of the Ammonites, and Makir son of
Ammiel from LoDebar, and Barzillai the Gileadite from
Rogelim brought bedding and bowls and articles
of pottery. They also brought wheat and barley,
flour and roasted grain, beans and lentils..."*
—2 Samuel 17:27–28 (NIV)

When King David was preparing to go into fierce battle against his son Absalom and his huge army, he was provided beans as part of the nourishment for his mighty warriors. The beans and other food must have been highly nutritious and energizing; the record informs us that David and his warriors defeated the army of Absalom in the forest of Ephraim.

Beans are mature seeds located within the pods of the legume plant. Other foods within the legume family include soybeans, lentils, chickpeas, and peas; peanuts are part of the family as well. Beans are low in calories, contain no cholesterol, and are extremely low in fat. The complex carbohydrates in beans provide sufficient energy for individuals maintaining an active lifestyle. Beans are also a gluten-free food.

Beans contain an ample amount of dietary fiber. The insoluble-fiber content creates bulk and moves food waste in a timely manner through the digestive tract and colon, significantly reducing the risk of colorectal disease and irritable bowel syndrome. The soluble fiber content decreases LDL (bad) cholesterol and triglycerides, lowering the risk of stroke and coronary heart disease. Beans are also loaded with protein, which supports the development and repair of tissue for normal growth and development, promotes and maintains strong muscle, and provides support to sustain the health of the immune system. Beans form the important complete protein when combined with grain foods such as brown rice, corn, or whole-wheat products. Beans were once commonly referred to as the poor man's meat due to their low cost and generous supply of protein.

The combination of fiber and protein slows the digestion and breakdown of food, which supports the slow release of sugar from the digestive tract into the bloodstream and contributes to the balancing of blood-sugar levels, great for managing diabetes. The small amount of sugar in beans also reduces the amount of insulin introduced into the bloodstream, which reduces the sensation of hunger, aiding weight loss goals.

Beans contain a generous supply of nutrients, including vitamins, minerals, and important phytonutrients. The phytonutrients in beans form a strong barrier against cell-damaging free radicals, reducing the risk of chronic disease; lignans reduces the risk of osteoporosis and increase cardiovascular health; and flavonoids significantly reduce the risk of cancer. Phytonutrients combine with beans containing the omega 3 fatty acid (navy and kidney beans) to reduce inflammation. Dark-colored beans, such as black beans, contain a higher level of phytonutrient and antioxidant strength.

Beans contain a variety of B vitamins, including folate for maintaining healthy arteries and protecting the development of the unborn fetus; B6 for creating new cells and helping the body break down protein; thiamin (B1) for proper nervous system and vital brain functions; and riboflavin (B2) for energy metabolism and healthy vision. Beans also contain important minerals, including calcium and copper for healthy bone structure; magnesium for relaxing arteries and improving blood and oxygen flow; potassium for healthy blood pressure and heart rate; iron for forming red blood cells and transporting oxygen to cells and tissue; manganese for healthy thyroid function and aiding the absorption of calcium; and zinc for healing wounds and maintaining sexual function.

To reduce the gas associated with beans, it's recommended that they be soaked for a minimum of twenty-four hours; soak at least overnight. Pour the water from the beans and rinse before cooking; check your beans before or after soaking for stones and poor quality beans. Soaking will also decrease the phytic acid contained in the beans. Phytic acid is a naturally occurring compound in beans, nuts, seeds, and grains that is well known to interfere with the body's absorption of important minerals, including calcium, magnesium, zinc, and iron (see Phytic Acid under Things You Should Know for soaking). Adding baking soda to beans will speed cooking time and reduce acidity but may decrease some of the nutrient value, particularly thiamin (B1), and may alter the delicious taste of the beans as well.

Peanuts, part of the bean family, are a significant part of the US diet and warrant a brief discussion. Peanuts are rich in heart-healthy monounsaturated fats and also contain a variety of important minerals, vitamins, and phytonutrients, particularly resveratrol, a phytonutrient contributing to cardiovascular health. Peanuts are also known to promote healthy brain function. According to The World's Healthiest Foods at www.whfoods.com, peanut antioxidant strength is equal to and better than that of some fruits and vegetables, and studies have shown that the rich mix of phytonutrients and other nutrients in peanuts reduces the risk of colorectal disease in men and women, and increases the health of the gallbladder by limiting stone formation. Peanuts contain significantly more fat and calories than other members of the bean family. Peanuts are a high allergen food; talk to your health-care professional if you notice allergic reactions to them or other foods.

Soybean and soybean-based foods receive mixed reviews. There is a tremendous amount of debate and disagreement associated with the consumption of soybeans and soybean-based foods. Some individuals celebrate soy products, and other individuals and health professionals label soybeans and soy-based products as toxic and a threat to good health. Anyone consuming or thinking of consuming this food should research it thoroughly; talk to your health-care professional as necessary concerning this food.

Following are profiles of commonly eaten legumes as provided by North Dakota State University's website at www.NDSU.edu, The World's Healthiest Foods at whfoods.com, and *Self* magazine's website at nutritiondata.self.com. In addition to nutrition facts, the glycemic index (GI) is given for each food.

Black Beans (1/2 cup) contain 114 calories, 0.5 grams total fat, 20.4 grams total carbohydrates, no cholesterol, 7.6 grams of protein, 7.5 grams of fiber, and no sugar; GI: Low.

Great Northern Beans (1/2 cup) contain 104 calories, 0.4 grams total fat, 18.7 grams total carbohydrates, no cholesterol, 7.4 grams of protein, 6.2 grams of fiber, and no sugar; GI: Low

Red Kidney Beans (1/2 cup) contain 112 calories, no fat, 20.2 grams of carbohydrates, no cholesterol, 7.7 grams of protein, 6.5 grams of fiber, and no sugar; GI: Low.

Navy Beans (1/2 cup) contain 127 calories, 0.5 grams total fat, 23.7 grams of carbohydrates, no cholesterol, 7.5 grams of protein, 9.6 grams of fiber, and 0.3 grams of sugar; GI: Low.

Pinto Beans (1/2 cup) contain 122 calories, 0.5 grams total fat, 22.4 grams of carbohydrates, no cholesterol, 7.7 grams of protein, 7.7 grams of fiber, and 0.3 grams of sugar; GI: Low.

Lentil Beans (1/2 cup) contain 115 calories, 0.4 grams total fat, 20 grams of carbohydrates, no cholesterol, 8.9 grams of protein, 7.8 grams of fiber, and 1.8 grams of sugar; GI: Low.

Black-Eyed Peas (1/2 cup) contain 100 calories, 0.4 grams total fat, 17.8 grams of carbohydrates, no cholesterol, 6.6 grams of protein, 5.6 grams of fiber, and 2.9 grams of sugar; GI: Low.

Peanuts (1/2 cup dry roasted) contain 431 calories, 37.8 grams total fat, 22 grams total carbohydrates, no cholesterol, 18 grams of protein, 6.7 grams of fiber, and 3 grams of sugar; GI: Low.

Food for Thought:

- Beans are a good source of protein, particularly when combined with other plant protein sources such as rice, corn, or wheat to form a complete protein.
- Dark-colored beans, such as black beans, contain higher levels of phytonutrient and antioxidant strength.
- Soak beans for the recommended time or at least overnight to lower gas and to remove some of the mineral-blocking phytic acid.
- Adding baking soda while preparing beans can reduce the B1 vitamin content.

- Peanut antioxidant strength is equal to and better than that of some fruits and vegetables.
- There is a tremendous amount of debate and disagreement associated with the consumption of soybeans and soybean-based foods. Some individuals celebrate soy products, and other individuals and health professionals label soybeans and soy-based products as toxic and a threat to good health; research and talk to your health-care provider if necessary.
- Beans are a gluten-free food.

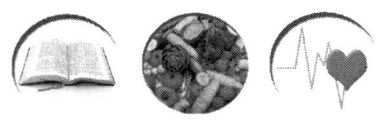

CHAPTER 5

WHOLE GRAINS AND THE WHEAT DEBATE

"Take wheat and barley, beans and lentils, millet and spelt; put them in a storage jar and use them to make bread for yourself..."
—EZEKIEL 4:9 (NIV)

Back in the times of the great prophet Ezekiel, grain was used to make highly nutritious and healthy food. With a small amount of individual grinding and necessary preparation, people were able to eat the entire grain and received a rich assortment of vitamins, minerals, phytochemicals, and other vital plant nutrients.

Grains come in the form of oats, wheat, rice, corn, barley, and others. Grains today are used to make various food products, including flour, bread, oatmeal, pasta, popular sweetened breakfast cereals, rice cakes, popcorn, and more. When identified as "whole grain," these products essentially contain the entire grain, including the bran, endosperm, and germ. In refined-grain products, the bran and germ are removed during the industrial milling process.

Many of the refined foods such as bread, cereal, rice, and others can be labeled "enriched," suggesting certain vitamins and minerals are added back to the product; however, these products are missing most of the valuable fiber, and about half of the important vitamins and minerals are still lost even after the enrichment process. Fiber, as you well know, is important in maintaining a healthy cardiovascular system due to its ability to regulate blood sugar and its contribution to lowering bad cholesterol in the blood. According to the Harvard School of Public Health, grain fiber also aids in reducing constipation and the risk of inflammatory diverticular disease (diverticulitis) in the colon and the consumption of brown rice and other whole grains instead of white rice can lower the risk of type 2 diabetes by as much as 36 percent.

Whole-grain products retain the valuable vitamins and minerals in the form of B vitamins, which are necessary for carbohydrate energy conversion, normal function of the muscles and nervous system, and red blood cell formation. The B vitamin, folate, is important for reducing neural tube defects during pregnancy and a variety of other life-sustaining functions, including the support of healthy blood vessels. Minerals are also a healthy part of whole grains, including manganese to facilitate the absorption of calcium and proper thyroid function and carbohydrate metabolism; iron to transport oxygen throughout the body and form red blood cells; magnesium to aid in the proper mineralization of healthy bones and support a healthy respiratory system; and selenium for its antioxidant support value; as well as copper, phosphorous, and zinc.

Be sure to always check the ingredient panel for the word "whole" in reference to the grain contained in the food you're considering. If the whole grain is there, you will have an effective source and quantity of fiber. Please do not confuse or associate "brown bread" with health; it's the grain quality of the bread or grain product and not the color that determines the nutrient value. Stay away from grain products that contain substances such as hydrogenated oils, bleached or bromated flour, aluminum of any kind, and other health-threatening ingredients.

According to the George Mateljan Foundation, whole wheat contains oxalates; persons with kidney or gallbladder issues, should talk to their health-care professional concerning this food. The foundation also suggests minimizing the consumption of baked snack foods containing wheat and sugar (crackers and cookies), and toasted grains such as toasted wheat cereals due to concerns related to cancer-causing acrylamides in these foods; talk to your health-care professional concerning these precautions.

The American Heart Association (AHA) indicates that the amount of grain an individual requires depends on age, gender, and calorie count; a two-thousand-calorie diet would likely include six to eight servings (ounces) of grain. The AHA also recommends individuals consume twenty-five grams of dietary fiber daily. Check your foods' packaging for the amount of fiber it contains; include the daily fiber received from other food sources as well, such as fruits and vegetables. Be sure to include an appropriate amount of water when consuming various grain fiber, many of which contain insoluble fiber that creates bulk; water aids proper passage through the digestive tract.

It's important to mention the heavily publicized and controversial wheat debate. Dr. William Davis, cardiologist and author of the popular *Wheat Belly* books, states that the modern wheat eaten today has toxic effects on the body, creating wheat allergies and a variety of health problems. This modern wheat, referred to as dwarf wheat and even "Frankenwheat" due to its alleged monstrous effects on health, is very different from the ancient wheat Ezekiel and even our grandparents ate. Dr. Davis states that this highly genetically modified wheat, invented to create greater global yield, is overloaded with gluten and contributes to heart disease, obesity, inflammation, diabetes, and other chronic health issues. Dr. Davis asserts that food products containing wheat flour, whole grain included, raise blood sugar significantly—more than table sugar.

Another concerned physician, Dr. Mark Hyman, family physician and best-selling author, supports the claims concerning the modern dwarf wheat, indicating that the super starch, amylopectin, in wheat flour and in popular baked goods containing this starch can cause serious spikes in blood-sugar levels. Dr. Hyman also states that the consumption of today's dwarf wheat is addictive and creates serious food cravings, contributing to insulin resistance (a precursor to type 2 diabetes) and weight gain.

As you might expect, there are health-care professionals and organizations that do not fully agree with the issues and concerns set forth concerning wheat. Eating any food is a personal decision; however, it's important to reveal the issues some health professionals have concerning this and other foods. It is increasingly important for individuals to be very aware of the foods they consume and any negative side effects. If you experience health issues including weight gain, blood sugar imbalance or other effects that may be associated with processed grain or other foods, please refrain from eating the specific food and talk to your health-care provider. Remember, you are in charge of protecting your health.

Individuals with Crohn's or celiac disease (an autoimmune disease that attacks the gluten protein and the small intestine) are very careful to avoid eating foods containing wheat, barley, rye, and other grains that contain the gluten protein. According to the Whole Grains Council, oats do not contain gluten unless contaminated by gluten grains during the growth or milling process. Certified gluten free oats are available for purchase. The council recommends that people with gluten sensitivity should have a conversation with their health-care provider to determine if the certified oats are safe for them. According to celiacdisease.about.com, grain products such as couscous, farro, and orzo are not gluten free foods.

Here are a few quick notes on some other gluten-free foods that some individuals may know little about. These pseudo-cereal grains resemble seeds and should be cooked for better digestibility; carefully follow any soaking preparation instructions.

- Buckwheat is a gluten-free pseudo-cereal that contains complete protein, plenty of soluble fiber for controlling blood sugar and supporting a healthy digestive tract, potassium for healthy blood pressure and heart rate, and an efficient supply of magnesium and phosphorous. It's used in several meals, including soup and salad dishes, and is also manufactured as flour.
- Quinoa is a gluten-free pseudo-cereal containing complete protein and important minerals, including manganese for increasing the utilization of antioxidants, phosphorous for proper cell function throughout the body, and ample potassium and magnesium. Quinoa is great in salads and other prepared dishes, sometimes replacing rice and other grains. It contains oxalates, so be careful if you're challenged with kidney disturbance; talk to your health-care provider.
- Amaranth is a gluten-free pseudo-cereal containing an ample supply of fiber and complete protein. It also contains efficient levels of phosphorous and potassium, and a supply of magnesium and calcium for bone health. Amaranth is used in many ways, such as in soups, salads, and baked goods, and it's also

produced as flour. It contains oxalates, so be careful if you have a kidney issue; talk to your health-care provider.

Food for Thought:

- For higher nutritional value, eat whole-grain foods as opposed to refined grains that tend to spike blood-sugar levels.
- The AHA recommends individuals consume twenty-five grams of dietary fiber daily; check food packages for fiber amount and include the daily fiber received from other food sources as well, such as fruits and vegetables.
- Individuals with Crohn's or celiac disorder should avoid grains containing the gluten protein; amaranth, buckwheat, and quinoa are not only gluten-free but also contain complete protein.
- Oats do not contain gluten unless contaminated with gluten grains during the growth, storage, or milling process; talk to your health-care provider concerning certified gluten-free oats.
- Grains products such as couscous, farro, and orzo are not gluten free foods.
- Avoid grain food products that contain aluminum, hydrogenated oils, bleached or bromated flour, or any other health-threatening ingredients; read the label.
- Drink appropriate amounts of water when eating high-fiber grain foods to keep waste moving through the digestive tract.
- Because of cancer concerns, exercise caution in overconsuming toasted wheat cereals and baked snack foods containing wheat and sugar.
- Talk to your health-care professional if you have any concerns about wheat or other foods.

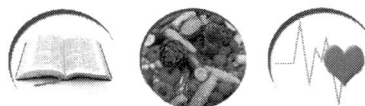

CHAPTER 6

POULTRY, FISH, AND MEAT

*"Your eye is the lamp of your body. When your eyes
are good, your whole body also is full of light."*
—Luke 11:34 (NIV)

Eating for nutrition rather than taste is the single most important thing you can do when it comes to food. However, spicy buffalo and hot wings, pizza loaded with dripping pepperoni, fried everything, and the triple-stacked burger are so woven into the fabric of today's eating culture that they've become an entrenched part of the Standard American Diet, shoving more nutritious food into a darkened background and past. This is not an indictment, but rather an observation of how much eating habits have changed in the past forty to fifty years. Maintain a well-balanced diet for sustainable health.

Poultry
Poultry consists of a variety of domestic birds that are used for food. Among the many varieties are chicken and turkey (the two most consumed) and duck—three of the most popular and commonly consumed birds.

Poultry provides several cuts of meat: the breast, wings, legs, and thighs are the more popular cuts. There are other parts of poultry that people consume, including the neck, back, tail, and internal organ meat. The breast meat is the most plentiful part of poultry, followed by the thigh, leg, and wing. Chicken is eaten four times as often as turkey in the United States and far more than duck. It's important to note that the amount of healthier omega 3 fatty acid is higher in chicken than turkey. It's also important to note that the World's Healthiest Foods at www.whfoods.com indicates there are 112 milligrams of sodium in four ounces of roasted turkey breast compared to 83 milligrams of sodium in four ounces of roasted chicken breast.

The breast meat of chicken and turkey is the healthiest part due to it containing less fat and calories than other parts of the bird. This is not true concerning duck breast meat, which is dark and contains a higher fat and calorie content than chicken or turkey breast; dark meat collects in the most often used muscle areas of poultry. To reduce the amount of fat consumed, eating the white meat of poultry would be a better choice. You've likely noticed the sizeable amount of fat contained under the skin, which should be removed before or after cooking if you're concerned with reducing overall fat intake; some leave the skin on during cooking only to retain moisture in the meat. Duck meat contains a comparatively higher fat content, even with the skin removed, and should be eaten sparingly.

Poultry contains a variety of nutrients, including protein, vitamins, and minerals, especially when pasture fed or fed nutritious grains. Included in the nutrients are B vitamins that support human cell development, proper nervous system function, carbohydrate and energy metabolism, and other important functions; chicken contains much more niacin (B3) than turkey for lowering LDL (bad) cholesterol and supporting cardiovascular and digestive health. Minerals include phosphorous for healthy cell function throughout the body; iron for transporting oxygen to cells and tissues and the formation of red blood cells; zinc for wound healing and normal fetal development; potassium for healthy blood vessels, heart rate, and blood pressure; magnesium for bone mineralization and respiratory health; and selenium (higher in turkey) for antioxidant support.

Protein is in rich supply to support the development and repair of tissue for normal growth and development, promote and maintain strong muscle, and provide support to sustain the health of the immune system. According to the United States Department of Agriculture (USDA), protein and calories are slightly higher in chicken than turkey. There are twenty-five grams of protein and 170 calories in three ounces of roasted chicken breast and twenty-four grams of protein and 160 calories in three ounces of roasted turkey breast.

For better nutrition, free-range or pasture-fed chicken or poultry is something to consider. Certified free-range and pasture-fed chickens that roam in natural sunlight and forage on natural plants and bugs are significantly more nutritious than caged birds raised under artificial light on pellet food. And if you have health concerns related to eating eggs, the eggs of certified free-range and pasture-fed hens contain significantly less cholesterol and saturated fat, and more than double the vitamin A, vitamin E, omega 3 fatty acids, and beta-carotene content, making them a better choice as well. There are multiple vitamins and minerals and 6.3 grams of high-quality, complete protein in a large egg; more than 50 percent of the protein resides in the egg white. A large boiled egg contains seventy-two calories. Look for the "no antibiotic" statement on the packaging of chicken and eggs. If you have cholesterol concerns, talk to your health-care professional concerning the safe number of eggs to consume per week.

Poultry's leaner protein can be used in a tremendous number of dishes. It's important to observe all of the handling, storage, and cooking precautions on the packaging. Poultry should be baked thoroughly to an internal temperature of at least 165 degrees Fahrenheit to avoid bacteria contamination and food-borne illness. Frying or grilling poultry at extremely high temperatures can create the development of carcinogenic compounds, including heterocyclic amines (HCA) and polycyclic aromatic hydrocarbons (PAH), which contribute to colon, breast, and prostate cancers.

Fish

Fish is a very interesting food, full of healthy omega 3 fatty acid, vitamins, and minerals. People tend to line up on one side of the aisle or the other concerning fish: They hate it, love it, or tolerate it. With the many nutrients contained in fish, it can play a major role in a healthy diet. Following are some things you should know.

Fish supports cardiovascular health with the aid of the omega 3 fatty acid, which helps to regulate heart rate and blood pressure, maintain the health of blood vessels to improve blood flow, and reduce the risk of arrhythmias (irregular heartbeats), which can be fatal. According to the Harvard School of Public Health, consuming one to two 3.5-ounce servings of fatty fish per week can reduce the risk of heart disease by one-third and is instrumental in the development of the brain and nervous system of the fetus during pregnancy.

Other research has revealed that fish high in omega 3 fatty acid, including mackerel, lake trout, herring, bluefin tuna, salmon, sardines, and albacore tuna, as well as a variety of fish that contain lesser amounts, can reduce the fats in blood and increase HDL (good) cholesterol, which provides additional support for heart health, reducing the risk of coronary disease and stroke. Eating fish is also linked to increased brain cognition as a result of its ability to improve blood flow, and it can also improve the weakened condition of skin and hair. The higher level of omega 3 fatty acids can also significantly reduce inflammation and chronic inflammatory diseases, such as arthritis.

Fish is a great source of quality protein and is low in saturated fat: three ounces of wild-caught salmon contains twenty-two to twenty-three grams of protein and 130 to 155 calories. Several other fish, such as cod, haddock, tuna, perch, and halibut, contain nineteen to twenty-six grams of protein and 90 to 130 calories in a three-ounce serving. Fish contains a wide variety of minerals, including selenium for anti-oxidant support, potassium for healthy blood vessels and increased blood flow, iodine for thyroid function, iron for transporting oxygen to cells and tissues, magnesium for healthy bones, zinc for healing wounds, phosphorous for healthy cell function throughout the body, and calcium for strong bones and teeth and proper blood clotting. Fish also contains B vitamins for energy metabolism and vitamin D for bone mineralization and the absorption of calcium.

It is strongly recommended that people refrain from eating large fish such as shark, swordfish, tilefish, and king mackerel because of high levels of toxins, including mercury and dioxins; dioxin is well known to increase the risk of cancer. Toxic compounds released into the rivers and waterways from industrial sites create many of the toxins that re-side in fish close to these shores. The larger fish in these waters tend to have significantly higher levels of toxins because of their size and their habit of eating smaller toxic fish. The age of the fish also impacts the level of toxin contained in its body. Farm-raised fish can contain toxins depending upon where the aquatic tanks are located in proximity to a polluting site. Dr. Melina Jampolis, CNN nutrition expert, recommends trimming the skin and fat from fish and cooking the fish (not fried) in a way that reduces the fat due to toxic chemicals being largely stored in the fat. If you're concerned about the safety of consuming specific fish, you can visit the Monterey Bay Aquarium Seafood Watch website at http://www.seafoodwatch.org/.

A great deal of discussion surrounds farm-raised versus wild-caught fish. Dr. Josh Axe, a noted clinical nutritionist, indicates that farm-raised fish are fed inferior foods, often made with ingredients such as chicken feces and other animal feces, and are also fed antibiotic chemicals and treated with strong pesticides to reduce disease and to keep the fish alive in the crowded conditions of the tank environment. Many health experts point out that, having very limited natural swimming space, farm-raised fish easily collect more unhealthy fat. Farm-raised fish also contain less usable omega 3 fatty acid and more inflammatory omega 6 fatty acid and have lower protein content than wild-caught fish. Tilapia, salmon, sea bass, catfish, and cod are some of the most common fish raised in aquatic farms; however, some of these fish are also caught in the wild.

On the other hand, true wild-caught fish from the deeper and purer parts of waters are leaner and contain higher levels of protein and usable omega 3 (great for healthy joints) than farm-raised fish. Dr. Axe also describes health concerns associated with the consumption of tilapia; you may want to conduct personal research within reliable and widely available information and talk to your health-care provider if concerned.

Shellfish, such as shrimp, crabs, lobsters, mussels, clams, and oysters, contain B vitamins and the minerals potassium, calcium, and iron; they're very high in zinc. Shellfish do not contain a high level of omega 3 fatty acid like some other fish. Shellfish are low in cholesterol, with the exception of shrimp, which contains twice as much as other seafood. Shellfish can trigger seafood allergies. Individuals following strict biblical guidelines eat only fish with fins and scales; foods such as catfish and shellfish are forbidden. However, you have to think and consider whether we're really meant to eat food that is sometimes dragged from up to fifteen thousand feet below the water surface, whose main function is to feed on death and waste while cleaning the ocean floor, and who also serve as important and vital food for other, larger marine animals; humankind was not meant to eat everything in the air, land, and sea.

Again, carefully follow handling, storage, and cooking instructions for fish. Bake fish to an internal temperature of 145 degrees Fahrenheit; avoid frying. It's important to note that the Mayo Clinic has shared the results of a large study that discovered regularly eating a single serving of fried fish per week increases the risk of heart failure by 50 percent; bake, broil, or grill fish at safe temperatures to avoid charring! You can visit various online sites, including the US Food and Drug Administration's guidelines at www.fda.gov/food/resourcesforyou/consumers/ ucm077331.htm, to gather additional information concerning the safe preparation of fish and other seafood.

Red Meat

Red meat, primarily beef, pork, and lamb, is a food source containing solid fats, but can be a source of protein. Healthier eating involves reducing the amount of solid fats consumed in favor of healthier food choices. Processed red meat such as bacon, sausage, and hot dogs also contribute to the cardiovascular health risk associated with the consumption of solid fats.

A Harvard University study concluded that daily consumption of red meat and processed red meat products has been linked to an increased risk of colorectal cancer. The cancer risk increases when the meat is grilled or fried at very high temperatures. Harvard University also concluded that intake of red meat and processed red meat at least five times per week boosts testosterone production, which significantly increases the risk of prostate cancer in men; red meat had a stronger correlation to prostate cancer than any other food group. And according to the Physicians Committee for Responsible Health, regular consumption of high fat foods such as meat boosts the production of the female hormone estrogen, significantly increasing the risk of estrogen-related breast cancer.

Red meat and some other foods contain high amounts of uric acid, which acidifies the body, creating crystallization in muscles and severe joint inflammation, contributing to gout and other health issues. Talk to your health-care professional if you have concerns or would like to learn more about this food.

Food for Thought:

- To reduce char and cancer-causing compounds, partially cook all meat products in the oven so they spend less time on the grill.
- Remove the skin and underlying fat before consuming poultry.
- Turkey contains a high level of sodium, and duck contains a very high level of fat; eat sparingly.
- Certified free-range and pasture-fed chickens, roaming in natural sunlight and foraging on natural plants and bugs, are significantly more nutritious than caged birds raised under artificial light and eating pellet food; this applies to eggs as well.
- Eat wild-caught fish as opposed to farm-raised fish; wild-caught fish provide better protein and omega-3, have less body fat, and are free of antibiotics and pesticides.

- Eat smaller fish as opposed to large fish that can contain significantly larger amounts of dangerous toxins.
- Trim the skin and fat from fish and cook the fish (not fried) in a way that reduces the fat due to toxic chemicals being largely stored in the fat.
- Eating fried fish once a week can increase the risk of heart failure by 50 percent.
- Rethink the need to consume bottom-dwelling seafood, such as catfish and shellfish, who serve as ecological vacuum cleaners; mankind was not meant to eat everything in the air, land, and sea that either flies, skydives, runs, creeps, crawls, hops, swims, or backstrokes.
- Due to high levels of saturated fats and increased risks of colorectal disease and prostate cancer, exercise caution in regularly consuming red meat and processed red meat products; red meat has the highest correlation to prostate cancer development than any food group.
- To reduce the risk of estrogen-related breast cancer, women should limit high fat foods such as meat, which produces high levels of estrogen.

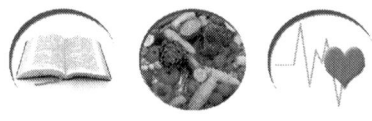

CHAPTER 7

HERBS AND SPICES

"He replied 'Because you have so little faith. I tell you the truth, if you have faith as small as a mustard seed, you can say to this mountain, 'move from here to there' and it will move. Nothing will be impossible for you."
—Matthew 17:20 (NIV)

Even the smallest things can bring about robust change. A mustard seed, one of the smallest of all the seeds, contains a huge, flavorful profile and is used primarily as a condiment and flavor addition around the world. There are tremendous health benefits to several of the small but mighty spices and herbs that wake up and add zest to an otherwise boring and bland dish. According to writers for the University of Michigan Hospital and Health Clinics at umich.edu, herbs and spices have different origins. Herbs, including basil and parsley, originate from plant leaves, while spices often originate from the seeds, berries, bark, or roots of plants.

There are several herbs and spices on the market today that add various flavor profiles to your favorite food dishes. In addition to their flavor, many of them provide health benefits such as vitamins, minerals, and phytonutrients, particularly antioxidant and anti-inflammatory nutrients. Herbs and spices are also great substitutes for traditional salt usage, reducing the risk of cardiovascular and blood-pressure health issues. Due to possible negative side effects involving toxicity in some instances, exercise caution in consuming large quantities of some herbs and spices, such as nutmeg, cinnamon, and ginger; research as appropriate and talk to your health-care provider if concerned.

Basil: Contains anti-inflammatory properties that reduce inflammation in the joints, reducing pain commonly associated with arthritis.

Black Pepper: The most common spice, black pepper has antioxidant and antibacterial compounds and is well known to improve digestion and act as a diuretic.

Cayenne: A hot and flavorful addition to food that has shown health benefits in the areas of improving circulation and supporting immune health to protect against colds and flu.

Cilantro: A rich source of vitamin K that helps in balancing blood calcium, blood clotting, and bone mineralization.

Cinnamon: A spice that has significant research to suggest it contains generous antioxidant compounds that reduce inflammation and also has the capacity to reduce blood glucose and triglyceride levels, in addition to treating nausea and stomach ulcers. Exercise caution in consuming large quantities due to possible negative side effects involving toxicity; research as appropriate and talk to your health-care provider if concerned.

Cumin: Can regulate blood-sugar levels and has beneficial effects in treating stomach disorders, such as ulcers.

Ginger: Well known to relieve motion sickness and nausea. It has been used to relieve some of the sickness associated with chemotherapy treatment. Caution: Excessive intake may prevent proper blood clotting; research as appropriate and talk to your health-care provider if concerned.

Mustard (Seeds): Contains antioxidants and anti-inflammatory properties, a wide variety of vitamins and minerals, and heart-healthy omega 3 fatty acids. Mustard seed is also known to have beneficial effects on respiratory health.

Nutmeg: A flavorful spice used in many dessert dishes. Contains anti-inflammatory properties that provide relief from inflammation and is known to reduce bacteria. Exercise caution in consuming large quantities due to possible negative side effects involving toxicity; research as appropriate and talk to your health-care provider if concerned.

Oregano: An herb that has anti-inflammatory and antioxidant compounds, which can relieve inflammation and add protections against chronic illness. Also contains antibacterial properties that can reduce the risk of food-borne illness.

Rosemary: An herb that contains a generous supply of antioxidant strength, reducing the risk of inflammation and cancer growth.

Sage: This Thanksgiving favorite contains a generous supply of vitamins, minerals, and phytonutrients, including vitamins A, C, E, and K, plus calcium, iron, magnesium, and potassium, to name a few. The phytonutrients in sage combine to create antioxidant protection and health benefits. Sage is also known to enhance memory.

Turmeric: Related to ginger, turmeric contains anti-inflammatory properties that can be used to reduce inflammation and improve joint health; also known to cleanse the liver and reduce the growth of cancer cells.

Thyme: A flavorful herb that contains ample antioxidant strength to reduce cancer-causing cellular damage and inflammation; it also boosts the immune system.

Food for Thought:

- For better health, use herbs and spices in place of salt.
- To avoid possible negative side effects, exercise caution in using some herbs and spices in large amounts, including cinnamon, nutmeg, and ginger; research and talk to your health-care provider if you have concerns.

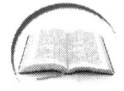 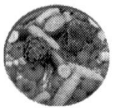 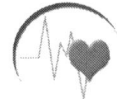

CHAPTER 8

WATER

"Worship the Lord your God and his blessing will be on your food and water. I will take away sickness from among you."
—Exodus 23:25 (NIV)

The scripture above clearly informs us that food and water are two inseparable sources of nourishment that are true blessings for our health and strength. Water is a resource that we can't live without. This is evidenced by the huge sums of money that are raised to ensure clean drinking water is made available to impoverished countries around the world. Without clean, fresh water, people would die in great numbers from disease and complete dehydration, proving to everyone that fresh water is a critical, life-sustaining substance.

The body and blood supply are composed of approximately 60 percent water. Clean, fresh water is a critical and absolutely essential element in maintaining health and proper hydration in the body. Water is vital for several bodily functions, including proper digestion; transporting nutrients to cells; controlling body temperature; eliminating toxins from the body; supporting proper function of the kidneys, liver, and other vital organs; reducing acidity; and retaining proper moisture in the body's tissues. Your brain, which is composed of approximately 75 percent water, functions much better and retains clarity when properly nourished with fresh water.

Choosing water over sugary soft drinks can significantly aid weight control and can provide proper hydration to your skin. Water combined with adequate fiber also helps the digestive tract maintain proper flow, reducing chronic constipation, hemorrhoids, and irritable bowel syndrome. Water from other sources, such as fresh fruits and vegetables, also contributes to proper hydration of the body.

Drinking plenty of clean, fresh water can actually reduce backaches, memory loss, acid reflux, and a variety of other common ailments. Water flushes uric acid (crystallization) buildup in the muscle caused by the consumption of red meat and other foods, which significantly contributes to incidents of low back and hip pain. Water also helps restore the pH balance in the stomach, reducing episodes of acid reflux. Cucumbers are excellent for this as well.

Sweetened fruit drinks or sugary sodas do not immediately satisfy the dehydration issue; these drinks go through the digestive system slower before going into the blood and cells for dehydration correction. Because there is no matter to breakdown, fresh water can be absorbed into the body within a few minutes if consumed with no food, and can begin to return the body to a state of hydration quickly provided enough water is consumed. However, it may be important for some to add fresh lemon or other healthy additives to water to enhance its taste—no problem, if that's what it takes for you to get an adequate supply of water.

The amount of water required is based on a number of factors, including environmental considerations such as climate and the level of exercise and physical activity a person engages in. People living in hot climates and/or engaging in moderate to intense exercise require more water. Products containing caffeine, such as coffee and tea, expel water from the body, causing a need for replacement; alcohol and refined sugar have the same dehydrating effect.

The daily recommendation for water intake is eight glasses or half your body weight in ounces. There is no challenge or debate to either of those recommendations; however, proper water intake is individual and should seek to satisfy the natural thirst impulse and to replace water lost daily through the skin, lungs, kidneys, and stools. Adequate water supply in the body can be reflected in the color of urine: a pale or light shade of yellow should be noticeable. Talk to your health-care provider if urine remains dark or brown when regularly consuming water.

A very important note concerning adequate hydration is that you must not fail to satisfy your natural thirst impulse. Continued avoidance of your natural thirst impulse can potentially place your body in a state of perpetual dehydration; adding to a variety of acidic, cardiovascular, muscular, and joint-health issues. It's also important not to overhydrate, which can create a serious sodium reduction in the blood, contributing to a variety of health conditions including severe muscle health issues. Some health professionals also warn against drinking extremely cold water due to its ability to slow digestion; room-temperature water is recommended. To avoid the dilution of the natural stomach acid required to digest your food, try to avoid drinking water or drink as little water as possible twenty to thirty minutes before, during, and after meals.

Drinking water the very first thing in the morning is a great way to rehydrate and rejuvenate your tissues and organs. According to livestrong.com, water in the morning also reduces the buildup of stomach acid from your nightly fast. A simple reminder: illness thrives in a dry body.

Food for Thought:

- Drink water upon rising in the morning to hydrate tissues and organs from the night fasting period; water provides initial morning alertness.
- Get adequate water supply daily for hydration, proper body function, and the removal of toxins.
- Drinking plenty of clean, fresh water can actually reduce back-aches, memory loss, acid reflux, and a variety of other common ailments.
- Don't ignore your natural thirst impulse, as doing so can add to a variety of acidic, cardiovascular, muscular, and joint-health issues.
- It's important not to overhydrate, which can create a serious sodium reduction in the blood, contributing to a variety of health conditions including severe muscle health issues.
- Consume water based on activity, climate, health status, and food-and-beverage consumption behaviors.
- Water-rich fruits and vegetables are great partners to fresh water for hydrating the body.
- Pale or light yellow urine indicate an adequate water supply in the body; talk to your health-care provider if urine remains dark or brown when regularly consuming water.
- Avoid drinking extremely cold water, as it slows digestion.
- To retain stomach acid strength to properly digest your food, avoid drinking water or drink as little as possible twenty to thirty minutes before, during, and after meals.

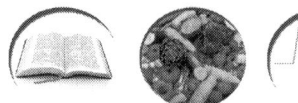

CHAPTER 9

MACRONUTRIENTS

Macronutrients

Macronutrients are comprised of three nutrients: carbohydrates, proteins, and fat, which provide calories and energy and are required in larger amounts to maintain healthy bodily function. Each macronutrient below contains an estimated daily intake range, which should be predicated on your personal health status and lifestyle. Carbohydrates represent the largest intake of foods.

Carbohydrates

Carbohydrates are classified as sugar, starch, and fiber and are broken into two basic categories: simple and complex. Simple carbohydrates are found in fruits, vegetables, milk, and milk products. Complex carbohydrates reside in starchy vegetables, such as potatoes, sweet potatoes, corn, beans, and peas, and in grain foods, including bread, pasta, cereal, and rice. Natural forms of complex carbohydrates as opposed to refined forms—in other words, whole-grain versus refined-grain foods—digest more slowly and consequently increase blood sugar at a slower rate and over a longer period of time, simultaneously decreasing insulin output and hunger.

Carbohydrates are converted into glucose (simple sugar) by the digestive system and are the body's primary source of fuel,

supplying all of the body's cell, tissue, and organ energy requirements. Carbohydrates are readily converted to and more usable
than fat or protein for energy. If there are insufficient carbohydrates available, the body will first convert fat and then protein
to carbohydrate for fuel; however, direct carbohydrate food is an
excellent and the most often used fuel source. Carbohydrates
contain four calories per gram. A small amount of glucose is converted to glycogen and stored in the body's liver for later energy
use and in the muscle for proper operation; the stored glycogen
is converted back to glucose as necessary. Unused or unconvert-
ed glucose is stored as fat.

Within the three classifications, sugar is considered a simple carbohydrate naturally contained in foods such as fruit (fructose), milk (lactose), honey (glucose and fructose), refined sugars such as table sugar
(sucrose), and vegetables. Starch is a complex carbohydrate naturally
contained in whole grains, starchy vegetables, beans, and peas. Fiber
is also a complex carbohydrate naturally found in whole grains, fruit,
vegetables, beans, peas, nuts, and seeds. Sugar and starch are the
fuel sources broken into simple sugars (glucose) during the digestion
process.

Fiber is the carbohydrate that is not broken down in the body. Fiber
moves through the digestive tract to aid the maintenance of digestive
health and is essential in the movement and elimination of waste through
the colon, reducing the risk of colorectal disease, diverticulitis (colon inflammation), and constipation. Fiber contributes to cardiovascular and
heart health by aiding in the reduction of LDL (bad) cholesterol in the
blood. Two basic types of fiber are soluble fiber (dissolves in water), which
forms a gel that moves food through the digestive tract much slower,
slowing the release of glucose into the bloodstream, and insoluble fiber

(does not dissolve in water), which creates bulk and pushes food through the digestive tract quicker. For example, apples and pears have a large quantity of soluble fiber, while green leafy vegetables and whole-grain foods have a large quantity of insoluble fiber.

Carbohydrates are also vital in supporting the proper function of the brain, kidneys, muscle, and nervous system. Again, to properly support these critical functions, it's tremendously important to eat a healthy variety of carbohydrates—in other words, fruit, vegetables, and whole grains as opposed to highly refined carbohydrate foods, such as refined bread, flour, sugar, polished rice, and so on. Exercise caution in consuming carbohydrate food products containing added sugar and sodium.

Many health professionals and organizations suggest that 45–65 percent of daily calories should come from carbohydrates. There is no debate; however, your carbohydrate intake should be compatible with your lifestyle and health status. Remember, carbohydrates create energy that's very useful for an active lifestyle, and they're required for normal bodily function. However, excess, unburned carbohydrate calories can interfere with weight-reduction goals, potentially contributing to other health issues such as obesity, diabetes, heart disease, and more. This is not intended to discourage consumption but rather to tailor consumption to your personal needs. Talk to your health-care professional to discuss your specific carbohydrate requirement and type based on your health status and lifestyle.

Protein

Protein is created by the body's building blocks, referred to as amino acids. According to Dr. Jethro Kloss, the brilliant author of *Back to Eden*, protein is required for a number of functions, including the growth and repair of tissue, maintaining the alkaline condition of body fluid, creating antibodies to aid in supporting a healthy immune system to defend the body against disease, and making enzymes and hormones. Protein is contained in every body cell and tissue, and the majority is in the muscles. Protein contains four calories per gram.

There are twenty-two identified amino acids in various combinations that form a variety of proteins. Nine are essential amino acids obtained from food sources, and these amino acids are the basis of a complete protein, and thirteen amino acids manufactured by the body that are classified as nonessential. All nine essential amino acids must be contained in the complete protein at a sufficient level for the protein to perform its important duties. Animal products such as meat, poultry, fish, milk, eggs, and a few plant food sources supply complete protein. Incomplete proteins by themselves don't have a sufficient level of essential amino-acid value to perform their tasks at an optimal level. Plant foods generally fall into this category; however, sesame and sunflower seeds, brazil nuts, quinoa, buckwheat, and amaranth are a few of the plant foods classified as complete proteins. Incomplete protein foods can be combined with other incomplete protein foods to establish a complete protein—for instance, beans eaten with grains such as rice, corn, or wheat, or natural (without additives) peanut butter eaten with whole-grain bread.

When eaten, protein is broken down in the digestive tract and forms individual amino acids, which are reassembled into specific proteins for the primary purpose of repairing damaged tissue or performing other identified duties when signaled. After performing a specific function, protein is not stored in the body like carbohydrates and fats, and because it's lost each day, it has to be replaced by the food we eat. However, it's important to note that although protein itself is not stored, excess amino acids, which form protein, are converted and stored as fat.

Eat a variety of plant proteins and supplement with other healthy complete proteins as necessary; exercise caution placing red meat at the top of the list—eat lean protein. Eating proper amounts of protein makes the body feel full, reducing hunger longer, which can contribute to weight maintenance and possibly stimulate slight weight loss.

Contrary to popular belief, protein itself does not burn fat; however, it may increase metabolism to burn a few additional calories. It's also important to point out that consuming protein alone will not build muscle; it's the exercise or training in conjunction with protein that builds muscle. It's also urban legend that individuals performing strenuous work require more protein; normal healthy muscles with the recommended protein intake combined with increased calories should provide sufficient energy in this instance.

As mentioned earlier, protein in the body can be used as fuel if necessary, but first the nitrogen contained in the protein must be removed for this to occur. This removal process creates highly acidic waste, which is eliminated in the urine, placing significant stress on the kidneys. Excess waste from the breakdown of protein has to be neutralized to prevent tissue damage, which draws calcium from the bones to act as a buffer, thereby weakening the bones. To maintain optimum health, consume only enough protein to meet recommended levels and to replace lost protein.

The daily recommendation for protein intake is forty-six grams for women and fifty-six grams for men. The Institute of Medicine recommends 10–35 percent of daily calories come from protein. Again, no debate; however, be careful with consuming excessive or high levels of protein based on the information provided. Talk to your health-care professional concerning the appropriate intake of this important macronutrient, particularly for children.

Some sources of protein include the following:

3 oz. chicken breast/24 grams	1 oz. sunflower seeds, almonds, and pistachios/6 grams
3 oz. wild caught salmon/22 grams	1 cup buckwheat/6 grams
½ cup dry roasted peanuts/18 grams	1 oz. pumpkin seeds and cashews, and 1 cup corn/5 grams
1 cup amaranth/9 grams	1 pomegranate/4.7 grams
6 oz. plain low fat yogurt/8.9 grams	1 medium baked potato/4.3 grams
1 cup green peas/8 grams	1 avocado/4 grams
1 cup quinoa/ 8 grams	1 cup broccoli/3 grams
½ cup red kidney beans, pinto beans, and black eyed peas/7.7 grams	1 medium zucchini/2.4 grams
½ cup black beans/7.6 grams	1 medium baked sweet potato/2.3 grams
½ cup navy beans/7.5 grams	½ cup asparagus/2.1 grams
½ cup great northern/7.4 grams	1 cup kale, green beans, and beets/2 grams
1 large egg/6.3 grams	1 medium wedge watermelon/1.74 grams

Fat

There are different types of dietary fats that the body is able to utilize and store. Dietary fat comes from the foods we eat and usually contains significant amounts of calories, which can contribute to weight gain and a variety of related health issues. However, fats do play positive roles, such as allowing fat-soluble vitamins A, D, E, and K to be absorbed into the body; serving as a reserve source of energy when necessary; and facilitating several metabolic functions in the body, such as insulating body organs, maintaining body temperature, and supporting healthy cell function. Fat contains nine calories per gram.

Today, it is critically important to understand the key difference between healthy and unhealthy fats. Fatty acids are contained in fats and have varying effects on health, largely dependent on the type and the amount consumed. Healthy fats are the monounsaturated fats that you've read about throughout this book and polyunsaturated fats, which include the popular omega 3 fatty acids that you also hear a lot about; these two healthier fats, when used as fuel, burn very efficiently. Fats that threaten the body's health are saturated fats and trans fats.

Monounsaturated fat found in a variety of foods and oils is shown to have a positive impact on lowering LDL (bad) cholesterol and protecting HDL (good) cholesterol levels, which contribute to cardiovascular and heart health and also provide support in controlling blood-sugar levels and reducing inflammation. Polyunsaturated fats found in fish, poultry, plant foods and oils, provide multiple benefits including its contribution to cardiovascular health. Unsaturated fats are liquid at room temperature.

Omega 3 fatty acids, a polyunsaturated fat and essential fatty acid that the body does not manufacture and therefore has to be obtained from food, provide a variety of health benefits, including acting as an anti-inflammatory agent when combined with other nutrients. Omega 3 also contributes to heart and cardiovascular health by having beneficial effects on triglyceride levels, blood pressure, and heartbeat. Food sources include healthy fatty fish such as salmon, sardines, mackerel, tuna, and trout. Omega 3 fatty acids are also contained in avocado, walnuts, kale, spinach, romaine lettuce, brussels sprouts, cauliflower, broccoli, green beans, strawberries, eggs from pasture-fed hens, low fat yogurt, and poultry. There is very little omega 3 contained in oils. It's important to note that the Mayo Clinic and other respected sources have revealed that recent studies are indicating that high levels of omega 3 fatty acids may be linked to an increased risk of prostate cancer. There are several documented conflicting opinions concerning the studies; if you're concerned, talk to your health-care professional.

Omega 6 fatty acids, a polyunsaturated fat and essential fatty acid that is not produced in the body and also has to be obtained from food, contributes to heart health and cholesterol control, but is well known to increase inflammation in the body and should be balanced with omega 3 fatty acids (healthy, wild-caught fatty fish and specific plant sources containing omega 3, such as romaine lettuce, can provide some balance). Sources with ample omega 6 include oils such as grape seed, sunflower, corn, soybean, sesame, walnut, peanut, and cottonseed; however, peanut and sunflower oils also contain an even higher level of omega 9 monounsaturated fat as well.

Omega 9 is a monounsaturated fatty acid that the body does produce in a very small quantity. This fatty acid is readily found in almond, avocado, peanut, sunflower, olive and high-oleic safflower oils. Foods containing omega 9 include avocado, olives, almonds, pecans, walnuts, peanuts, pistachios, eggs, and skinless poultry. The presence of omega 9 reduces LDL (bad) cholesterol and increases HDL (good) cholesterol, which limits plaque buildup in the arteries, reducing the risk of coronary heart disease and stroke.

On the other hand, unhealthy, saturated fats place a significant burden on the body. Saturated fats are found primarily in animal sources and contribute to the increase of blood cholesterol, particularly LDL (bad) cholesterol, which can have a negative impact on cardiovascular and heart health. Saturated fat is contained in red meat, poultry with skin, palm and coconut oil, cheese, butter, and high-fat dairy products. Unhealthy fats, particularly red meat and processed red meat, also contribute to colorectal disease, breast and prostate cancer, obesity, and other health issues.

Trans Fat

Trans fat is primarily the result of the artificial process of hydrogenating or partially hydrogenating oils to make them solid to increase their shelf life and improve their cooking quality. Trans fat contributes to the increase of LDL (bad) cholesterol and decrease of HDL (good) cholesterol in the blood, contributing to the blockage of blood vessels and coronary artery disease. Trans fat is contained primarily in fried foods, commercial bakery products, margarine and vegetable shortening, and in food products that contain these hydrogenated substances. Carefully read the packaging on products such as microwave popcorn, potato chips, and premixed baking products. Trans fats and saturated fats are solid at room temperature; think about it.

It's also important to know what's contained in some fat-free foods. When the fat is removed, some products often contain added sugar, sodium, or a mixture of food additives to increase the taste. Again, read the labels and look for products that contain fewer and healthier ingredients. Talk to your health-care provider concerning these products in relationship to your health status!

Eat healthy fats. According to clevelandclinic.org and other information sites, total fat intake should range between 20 and 35 percent of calories, and saturated fats should be limited to less than 10 percent of calories; avoid trans fat completely.

Food for Thought:

- Excess protein, when broken down, can be damaging to kidneys, bones, and body tissue.
- Be careful of myths surrounding protein, for example, protein alone builds muscles, more protein is required to perform strenuous work, and protein burns fat.
- Eat adequate complete protein daily through plant or healthier animal and animal-product sources, such as non/low-fat yogurt.
- Eat healthier monounsaturated and polyunsaturated fats and fewer saturated fats; avoid trans fats entirely.
- Unhealthy saturated fats contribute to breast and prostate cancer, colorectal disease, obesity, and other health issues.
- Mayo Clinic and other respected sources have revealed that recent studies are indicating that high levels of omega 3 fatty acids may be linked to an increased risk of prostate cancer. There are several documented conflicting opinions concerning the studies; if you're concerned, talk to your health-care provider
- For better energy production and utilization and to avoid spikes in blood sugar, eat healthier and natural sugar and starch

carbohydrates, for example, fruits, vegetables, whole grains, and so on as opposed to refined carbohydrates.

- Be sure to get enough daily fiber to maintain healthy blood-sugar levels and aid digestion.

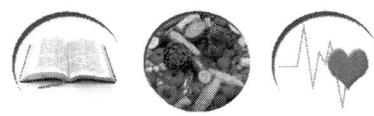

CHAPTER 10

MICRONUTRIENTS

Micronutrients

Micronutrients are commonly referred to as vitamins and minerals, and the name suggests that your body requires a lesser amount than macronutrients. Vitamins and minerals are critically important in the health and function of the entire body. Deficiencies in any of these critical micronutrients can have a devastating and lasting impact on your health. For purposes of identification and description, phytonutrients are also placed in this category.

Vitamins

Vitamins are organic substances that are essential for the proper function, growth, and health of the body. Vitamins can be obtained from various sources, including the plant foods we eat, meat from animals that consume vitamin-rich vegetation, and manufactured supplements.

Vitamins are separated into two groups: water soluble and fat soluble. Water-soluble vitamins, including B complex vitamins and vitamin C, are absorbed in the body through the body's water content. These vitamins are not stored in the body and their excess is eliminated in the urine, causing need for replenishment. Fat-soluble vitamins, including vitamins A, D, E, and K, are absorbed in the body through the body's fat content. These vitamins are stored in the body, and because they're stored, may have ill effects if stored in excess;

however, they must be replenished as the body's storage is depleted. All vitamins designated for a specific function must be present. A diet rich in healthy natural foods, such as fruits, vegetables, whole grains, beans, nuts and seeds, and lean protein, should supply the requisite vitamin requirements. Talk to your health-care professional concerning personal vitamin needs and whether you're taking any vitamins in excess of recommended levels.

Listed below are all known vitamins and their related health benefits.

Vitamin A: Promotes growth and repair of body tissue; supports a healthy immune system; contributes to healthy skin and hair; has recently been shown to reduce the risk of lung and oral-cavity cancers; and is critical to healthy vision, including night vision and reducing age-related vision loss (macular degeneration). Excellent sources include apples, cantaloupe, grapefruit, tomatoes, watermelon, carrots, broccoli, collard greens, kale, peas, romaine lettuce, sweet potatoes, cheese, eggs, and tuna.

Vitamin B1 (thiamin): Required for the normal function of the heart, nervous system, and muscles, and also needed for carbohydrate energy conversion. Excellent sources include avocado, grapefruit, oranges, pineapple, pomegranate, asparagus, brussels sprouts, butternut squash, corn, french green beans, lima beans, okra, green peas, sweet potatoes, brazil nuts, cashews, chestnuts, flaxseed, hazelnuts, macadamia nuts, oats, peanuts, pecans, pistachios, brown rice, rye, wheat, beans, peas, milk, salmon, and tuna.

Vitamin B2 (riboflavin): Important for vision; carbohydrate energy conversion; and proper nervous system, heart, and muscle function. Excellent sources include avocado, grapes, mango, pomegranate, artichoke, asparagus, brussels sprouts, french green beans, lima beans, mushrooms, green peas, pumpkin, winter squash, sweet potatoes, almonds, buckwheat, chestnuts, oats, rye, wheat, soybeans, cheese, cottage cheese, cream cheese, chicken, eggs, herring, perch, pollack, salmon, sardines, tuna, goat cheese, turkey, and low-fat yogurt.

Vitamin B3 (niacin): Excellent for lowering LDL (bad) cholesterol and raising HDL (good) cholesterol, supports healthy digestive and nervous systems and energy metabolism, increases circulation, protects cognitive capacity, and maintains healthy skin. Excellent sources include avocado, bananas, black berries, dates, mango, nectarines, peaches, pineapples, plums, pomegranate, raspberries, strawberries, tomatoes, watermelon, artichoke, asparagus, brussels sprouts, carrots, collard greens, corn, eggplant, french green beans, kale, lima beans, mushrooms, okra, onions, green peas, potatoes, pumpkin, squash, sweet potatoes, almonds, barley, buckwheat, chestnuts, hazelnuts, macadamia nuts, oats, peanuts, pumpkin seeds, brown rice, rye, sunflower seeds, wheat, beans, peas, cod, herring, perch, pollack, salmon, sardines, tuna, turkey, chicken, and duck.

Vitamin B5 (pantothenic acid): Aids in normal growth and development and in making hormones, such as adrenalin, and supports energy metabolism. Excellent sources include avocado, dates, grapefruit, pomegranate, watermelon, corn, lima beans, mushrooms, squash, sweet potatoes, buckwheat, oats, rye, sunflower seeds, wheat, beans, peas, chicken, milk, eggs, herring, perch, salmon, sardines, tuna, turkey, duck, and low-fat yogurt.

Vitamin B6 (pyridoxine): Important for protein metabolism and normal brain and nerve function, relaxes blood vessels, and creates red blood cells. Excellent sources include apples, avocado, berries, cherries, dates, figs, grapefruit, grapes, lemons, mango, oranges, pineapple, pomegranate, raisins, tomatoes, watermelon, artichoke, asparagus, broccoli, brussels sprouts, carrots, cauliflower, celery, collard greens, corn, kale, lima beans, okra, onions, green peas, potatoes, pumpkin, romaine lettuce, squash, sweet potatoes, barley, buckwheat, cashews, chestnuts, hazelnuts, oats, pistachios, brown rice, rye, sunflower seeds, walnuts, wheat, beans, peas, chicken, eggs, cod, herring, perch, pollack, salmon, sardines, tuna, and low-fat yogurt.

Vitamin B7 (biotin): Aids the proper function of the nervous system, provides health to muscle tissue, contributes to healthy skin and hair, and supports the body in producing energy. According to WebMD, a deficiency may contribute to hair thinning, tingling of arms and legs, and scaly rash around eyes, nose, and mouth. Food sources include avocado, bananas, raspberries, broccoli, cauliflower, salmon, egg yolks (egg whites decrease yolks' biotin value), and whole wheat bread.

Vitamin B-9 (Folate): Required to make DNA, aids the body in making red blood cells, reduces the risk of neural tube defects during pregnancy, maintains healthy arteries, and supports nervous system function. Excellent sources include avocado, bananas, berries, dates, mango, oranges, papaya, pineapple, pomegranate, artichoke, asparagus, beets, broccoli, brussels sprouts, cauliflower, celery, collard greens, corn, french green beans, lima beans, okra, green peas, potatoes, spinach, squash, buckwheat, chestnuts, hazelnuts, oats, peanuts, rye, sunflower seeds, walnuts, wheat, beans, peas, eggs, salmon, soy milk, and low-fat yogurt,

Vitamin B12: Important in maintaining a healthy nervous system, supporting the breakdown of fatty acids and amino acids, and making new red blood cells. According to the National Institute of Health, deficiency in vitamin B-12 can result in tingling in the arms and legs, loss of balance, weakness, and anemia. Excellent sources include milk, eggs, cod, herring, perch, pollack, salmon, sardines, tuna, and low-fat yogurt.

Vitamin C (ascorbic acid): Vitamin C is necessary for proper growth and development. It aids the body in absorbing iron; supports the proper healing of wounds; acts as a water-soluble antioxidant to arrest the development of free radicals, reducing the risk of chronic diseases such as cancer; boosts the immune system; prevents infections; and helps to create collagen, which holds the body's cells together. Smokers lose vitamin C and benefit greatly from vitamin C intake. Exposing vitamin C to cooking and long storage periods can reduce vitamin C content. The Institute of Medicine recommends a daily allowance of 90 mg for men and 75 mg for women. Excellent sources include grapefruit, kiwifruit, lemons, mango, oranges, papaya, pineapple, strawberry, broccoli, brussels sprouts, red and green bell peppers, cantaloupe, cauliflower, romaine lettuce, collard greens, and kale.

Vitamin D: Manufactured inside the body with the aid of the skin's exposure to natural sunlight. Aids in strengthening bones by assisting the body in absorbing calcium, helps to maintain proper levels of calcium and phosphorous in the blood, and helps to retain minerals in the bones. Excellent food sources include cod liver oil, salmon (3 ounces provides the daily requirement), tuna, cod, herring, sardines, eggs, fortified milk, cheese, cream cheese, sour cream, and yogurt.

Vitamin E: Acts as a fat-soluble antioxidant in protecting the body from cancer-causing free-radical damage. Vitamin E also engineers glucose energy release, supports normal growth and development, supports healthy red blood cells and the immune system. Vitamin E is well known to promote healthy skin and hair. Excellent sources include avocado, berries, cranberries, kiwifruit, mango, nectarines, papaya, peaches, pomegranate, asparagus, broccoli, butternut squash, pumpkin, sweet potatoes, almonds, brazil nuts, hazelnuts, peanuts, pine nuts, sunflower seeds, wheat, pinto beans, eggs, herring, and sardines. Men, talk to your health-care provider prior to taking high doses of vitamin E supplements due to a possible increase in prostate-cancer risk.

Vitamin K: Required for normal blood clotting, balancing blood calcium levels to reduce the risk of artery calcification, and helping to maintain bone density to reduce the risk of osteoporosis. Excellent sources include broccoli, brussels sprouts, collard greens, kale, romaine lettuce, and spinach. Vitamin K may interfere with blood thinning medication; talk to your health-care provider if this applies to you.

Minerals

Minerals are very important in supporting the health and maintenance of the body and contribute significantly to many of the body's primary functions and processes. Minerals are heavily involved in the proper function of the muscles and nervous system, maintaining water balance, and strengthening bones. The body does not manufacture minerals, so they are obtained from the food supply. The body's need for minerals is very small when compared to the macronutrients carbohydrates, protein, and fat. Minerals also tend to maintain their nutrient value in food, even after cooking.

Minerals are broken into two categories based on the amount required by the body: macrominerals and microminerals (also known as trace minerals). Macrominerals are required in larger amounts and trace minerals in smaller amounts.

Macrominerals are calcium, potassium, magnesium, sodium, sulfur, phosphorous, and chloride. Trace minerals required in smaller amounts include manganese, iodine, iron, copper, selenium, zinc, chromium, fluorine, and molybdenum. Calcium and phosphorous comprise the vast majority of the mineral supply in the bones; calcium alone accounts for approximately half.

Macrominerals

Calcium: Is essential for developing and maintaining strong bones and teeth, helps to reduce the risk of osteoporosis, supports vitamin absorption, aids in the proper clotting of blood, supports proper nerve and muscle function, and is instrumental in the absorption of iron. The presence of vitamin D helps the body to absorb calcium. The National Institute of Health recommends a daily allowance of 1,000 mg for adults, 1,300 mg for teens, 1,200 mg for women ages fifty-one to seventy, and 1,200 mg for ages seventy-one and over.

Excellent sources of calcium include the following

low fat plain yogurt (400mg/cup)	almonds (75mg/1 ounce)
sardines (325mg/3 ounces canned)	papaya (73mg/one medium)
non-fat milk (306mg/cup)	sweet potatoes (68mg/one baked)
cheddar cheese (303mg/1W.5 ounces)	celery (63mg/cup cooked)
collard greens (266mg/cup cooked)	broccoli (62mg/cup cooked)
black eyed peas (211mg/cup cooked)	oranges (60mg/one medium)
romaine lettuce (206mg/head)	dates (57mg/cup)
american cheese (195mg/1 ounce)	brussels sprouts (56mg/cup cooked)
oatmeal (187mg/cup)	green peas (43mg/cup cooked)
salmon (181mg/3 ounces canned)	blackberries (42mg/cup)
bok choy (158mg/cup)	pinto beans (39mg/half cup cooked)

baked beans (154mg/cup canned)	pumpkin (37mg/cup cooked)
okra (123mg/cup cooked)	cabbage (36mg/half cup cooked)
spinach (122mg/half cup cooked)	hazelnuts (32mg/1 ounce)
cheerios (114mg/cup)	pistachios (31mg/1 ounce)
french beans (112mg/cup cooked)	whole wheat bread (30mg/slice)
sour cream (104mg/four ounces)	walnuts (28mg/1 ounce)
non-fat cream cheese (98mg/ ounce)	eggs (25mg/one large boiled)
kale (90mg/cup raw)	sunflower seeds (20mg/1 ounce)
white beans (81mg/cup cooked)	apples (11mg/one medium)

Phosphorous: Supports the production of protein, is critical in the proper function of cells throughout the body, promotes strong bones and teeth, properly transports fatty acids to required areas of the body, and maintains the acid and alkaline fluid balance. Excellent sources are avocado, dates, pomegranate, asparagus, broccoli, brussels sprouts, butternut squash, corn, lima beans, okra, green peas, potatoes, pumpkin, sweet potatoes, nuts and seeds, barley, brown rice, rye, wheat, beans, peas, cheese, milk, cottage cheese, cream cheese, chicken, eggs, fish, turkey, sour cream, and yogurt.

Potassium: The third most abundant mineral in the body maintains the electrolyte and water balance in blood and tissue; works closely with other electrolytes, including sodium, to maintain heart health; regulates blood pressure and heart rate; supports healthy muscle contraction and proper function of the nervous system; and is involved in the production of protein. Too little or too much potassium in the blood may result in muscle weakness and fatigue; 4,700 mg per day are recommended. Excellent sources include just about all fruit, but potassium is abundant in avocado, bananas, dates, citrus fruit, and pomegranate. Rich vegetable sources include potatoes, sweet potatoes, and tomatoes. Other sources include brussels sprouts, butternut squash, celery, lima beans, green peas, pumpkin, winter squash, oats, rye, wheat, beans, peas, milk, salmon, sardines, and yogurt.

Magnesium: Supports the proper function of muscles and the nervous system; aids the body in creating protein, supports normal heart rhythm and blood pressure, provides support for a healthy immune system and respiratory health, and is important in proper bone mineralization to maintain a healthy bone structure. Excellent sources include avocado, bananas, blackberries, dates, pomegranate, watermelon, butternut squash, corn, lima beans, okra, green peas, potatoes, sweet potatoes, nuts and seeds, oats, rye, brown rice, sunflower seeds, wheat, beans, peas, tuna, cod, sardines, and low-fat yogurt.

Sodium: Sodium is contained primarily in body fluid outside of the cells, and the remainder resides in the bones. Works with potassium to maintain fluid and electrolyte balance in the cell, supports the normal function of muscles and the nervous system, and maintains acid and alkaline balance. Sources include avocado, cantaloupe, olives, pomegranate, tomatoes, beets, broccoli, celery, sweet potatoes, kale, romaine lettuce, spinach, cheese, cottage cheese, cream cheese, chicken, milk, eggs, fish, turkey, and yogurt.

Sulfur: Sulfur is an important mineral contained in every cell in the body and is essential for the proper function of insulin in the body. It plays an important role in the proper function of enzymes; supports detoxification; supports the structure and activity of proteins; and aids in maintaining healthy skin, hair and nails. Sources include eggs, milk, fish, poultry, onions, garlic, cabbage, asparagus, kale, and legumes.

Chloride: Chloride is an electrolyte mineral contained throughout the body in cells, fluid, and blood, mingling with potassium, sodium, and water to properly balance body fluids in and around cells. Also supports acid-alkaline balance and healthy kidney, nerve, and muscle function; is important in expelling excess fluid from the body; helps to properly move carbon dioxide from the body; and combines with hydrogen in the stomach to form normal stomach acids required to properly digest food. Sources include olives, tomatoes, cucumbers, carrots, celery, lettuce, kelp (seaweed), rye, and pineapple.

Microminerals (Trace Minerals)

Manganese: Manganese has several important functions, including ensuring proper function of the thyroid, aiding in the absorption of calcium, helping the body metabolize carbohydrates to maintain healthy blood-sugar levels, supporting the body in the effective use of antioxidants, and creating essential enzymes for building strong bones. Excellent sources include spinach, pineapple, oats, brown rice, pumpkin seeds, rye, collard greens, strawberries, raspberries, sweet potatoes, walnuts, navy beans, romaine lettuce, cabbage, garlic, kale, and cinnamon.

Iodine: Iodine is critically important for the normal function of the thyroid gland. Iodine helps to regulate growth and development and normal metabolism within the body, such as supporting food conversion to energy. A deficiency can create goiter growth in the neck region and slight bulging of the eyes. Rich sources of iodine are in seaweeds such as kelp and dulse. Iodine is also contained in sardines, tuna, salmon, haddock, spinach, garlic, summer squash, lima beans, turnip greens, and milk.

Iron: Iron has many functions in the body. Iron is an important component of the hemoglobin protein, which transports oxygen in the blood supply to tissues and organs throughout the body. Iron is also important in the formation and function of red blood cells, and energy metabolism. Iron is an important mineral for muscle health and proper function. Iron is a mineral that has to be balanced; too little creates anemia, and too much creates serious health issues amounting to iron poisoning. Women and children require a slightly larger daily amount of iron than men—8 mg for men, 15–18 mg for women, and 30 mg for pregnant women (women over fifty years of age require less than 10 mg). Depending upon age, children require 8–10 mg. Iron is contained in green leafy vegetables, yellow vegetables, potatoes, beans, lentils, green beans, raisins, and meat.

Copper: Copper is necessary for the proper absorption and use of iron and is important in the formation of red blood cells. Copper is also used for the production of energy and aids in strengthening connective tissue and bones. Copper relieves inflammation associated with arthritis, supports a healthy immune system, acts as a shield against nerve damage, and reduces LDL (bad) cholesterol in the blood. Sources of copper include avocado, black berries, dates, mango, pomegranate, kale, green peas, potatoes, pumpkin, almonds, brazil nuts, cashews, chestnuts, hazelnuts, oats, pecans, pistachios, pumpkin seeds, rye, sunflower seeds, walnuts, wheat, and cheese.

Selenium: Selenium is a companion to vitamin E in adding antioxidant and immune strength to the body. Selenium is a phytonutrient that significantly supports the battle against cancer and also behaves as an anti-inflammatory agent. Selenium provides support for the health of the thyroid gland. Sources of selenium include brazil nuts, asparagus, mushrooms, cod, tuna, salmon, sardines, turkey, chicken, eggs, milk, spinach, brown rice, sunflower seeds, broccoli, garlic, and cabbage. Men, talk to your health-care provider prior to taking high doses of selenium supplements due to a possible increase in prostate-cancer risk.

Zinc: Zinc is found in many foods and resides primarily in the muscles and bones in the body. Zinc is essential for normal growth and development and sustaining a strong immune system. It has been found to be necessary in the proper healing of wounds. Zinc is also important for producing protein and the proper conversion of carbohydrates to energy. Additionally, zinc is important for the sense of taste and smell, the normal development of a fetus, supporting sperm production, promoting the utilization of vitamin A, and contributing to healthy skin. According to the Consumer Health Organization of Canada at www.consumerhealth.org, zinc can reduce the toxic effect of certain metals in the body, such as iron and cadmium. Sources of zinc include oysters, avocado, pomegranate, green peas, oats, rye, sunflower seeds, pumpkin seeds, pecans, pine nuts, almonds, cashews, brazil nuts, beans, milk, cheese, eggs, yogurt, chicken, turkey, sardines, and meat.

Chromium: Chromium is an important mineral that primarily aids insulin in regulating blood-sugar levels in the body and helps in converting glucose into energy. Sources of chromium include apples, bananas, broccoli, tomatoes, onions, green beans, romaine lettuce, oats, barley, brown rice, milk, eggs, and chicken. Chromium is also found in brewer's yeast.

Fluorine: Fluorine is a beneficial trace mineral acting as fluoride that helps protect teeth from decay and has been shown to strengthen bones against osteoporosis. Sources include tea, saltwater fish (e.g., ocean perch, tuna, cod, snapper, sardines, halibut, mackerel, etc.), and fluoridated water.

Molybdenum: Molybdenums' presence in specific food sources is determined by soil conditions; soil deficient in molybdenum is unable to support plants grown in such soil. Molybdenum metabolizes carbohydrates into energy; detoxifies sulfites, which are often used as preservatives at salad bars and in wine; and aids in the utilization of iron. Sources include green beans, cauliflower, potatoes, spinach, beans, lentils, peas, oats, buckwheat, and brewer's yeast.

Phytonutrients

There are several thousand compounds or chemicals in plants that offer a wide range of protection for the plant, including protection from insects, disease, ultraviolet exposure, and other vulnerabilities. Fruits and vegetables are the primary recipients of these phytonutrients; however, they're contained in other plant foods as well, such as whole grains, nuts, and beans.

Phytonutrients (also known as phytochemicals) are not classified as essential for the preservation of life; however, they do offer many health benefits, including acting as antioxidants and anti-inflammatory agents in the body, and are well known to slow the aging process and contributing to healthy cell functions and increased organ and tissue health. The various identified phytonutrients in plants provide specific protections against chronic diseases, such as cancer, asthma, arthritis, cardiovascular and heart disease, and age-related eye disease (such as cataracts), and are well known to slow the aging process and provide a boost to the immune system.

Phytonutrients also provide the beautiful and rich colors in plant foods and are Mother Nature's resident painter, providing the red colors in strawberries, watermelon, tomatoes, red bell peppers, beets, and others; the orange and yellow colors in peaches, cantaloupe, oranges, carrots, sweet potatoes, pumpkin, squash, and others sharing this hue; the deep green color in kale, spinach, collard greens, romaine lettuce, and other green vegetables; the blue and purple colors in blueberries, blackberries, eggplant, and plums; and the white color of onion, cauliflower, and garlic. That's why it's so important to eat the "rainbow" of colors for sustainable health and nutrition.

The categories below are some of the more commonly known phytochemical agents, some of which may belong to the same family.

Beta-carotene: The majority converts to vitamin A in the body. It boosts the immune system and discourages free-radical development. It is found in the yellow and orange foods as well as the green leafy vegetables, including cantaloupe, pumpkin, sweet potatoes, carrots, apricots, peaches, squash, collard greens, kale, romaine lettuce, spinach, broccoli, and others.

Lycopene: Reduces the incidence of cancer, including prostate cancer, and supports heart health. Lycopene is found in red-colored foods, including tomatoes and tomato products, strawberries, cherries, red bell pepper, watermelon, and grapefruit.

Lutein: Contributes to the health of the eyes and heart, and reduces the risk of cancer. It is found in green foods, including collard greens, kale, spinach, romaine lettuce, broccoli, and brussels sprouts, and can also be found in bright-colored foods, including pineapple, bananas, pears, lemons, and avocados.

Resveratrol: Contributes to heart health by producing nitric oxide, which relaxes blood vessels to increase blood flow and reduce pressure in the blood; also reduces LDL (bad) cholesterol. In lab studies, resveratrol has demonstrated signs of slowing the growth of cancerous and inflammatory cells. Studies have been largely confined to the laboratory; more human studies are required to test the effectiveness of this phytonutrient in humans. Sources are red wine, red grapes and grape juice products, and peanuts.

Anthocyanidins: Contribute to the health of the blood vessels and protect against cancer and neurodegenerative disease, such as Alzheimer's disease, Anthocyanidins are found in red-colored foods such as strawberries, raspberries, cranberries, red onion, red potatoes, and radishes, and in blue and purple foods such as blackberries, blueberries, plums, and grapes.

Flavonols: Part of the flavonoid family that increases antioxidant capacity to neutralize cell-damaging free-radical activity and provides significant anti-inflammatory protections. Flavonols are found in apples, apricots, blueberries, green beans, broccoli, and yellow onions.

Food for Thought

- Vitamins, minerals, and phytonutrients together are vital to overall health and should be present in the body in proper levels to minimize health issues associated with their individual deficiencies; review favorite fruits and vegetables for the vitamin and mineral supply you may be lacking.
- Phytonutrients (also known as phytochemicals) are not classified as essential for the preservation of life; however, they do offer many health benefits, including acting as antioxidants and anti-inflammatory agents in the body, and are well known to slow the aging process.
- Vitamin C is recognized as one of the most important phytonutrients in supporting the immune system, significantly reducing

free-radical development and limiting the growth and spread of infection. Generous supplies are found not only in oranges, but also in broccoli, red bell peppers, and kale.

- Vitamin B12 deficiency can result in loss of balance, weakness, anemia, and tingling in the arms and legs.
- Potassium is vital for blood pressure and heart rate, and phosphorous is a multitasking mineral that is irreplaceable for the proper function of human cells throughout the body and for bone health. Too much or too little potassium can result in weakness and fatigue.
- Chromium is an important mineral that primarily aids insulin in regulating blood-sugar levels in the body and helps in converting glucose into energy. Apples are a great source.
- Zinc can reduce the toxic effect of certain metals in the body, such as iron and cadmium.
- Men, talk to your health-care provider prior to taking high doses of vitamin E and selenium supplements due to a possible increase in prostate-cancer risk.
- Talk to your health-care professional concerning personal vitamin needs and whether you're taking any vitamins in excess of recommended levels.

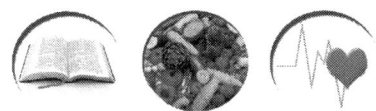

CHAPTER 11

SOME THINGS YOU SHOULD KNOW

Salt (sodium)

Salt is composed of 40 percent sodium and 60 percent chloride, combining to create sodium chloride, or table salt. Sodium chloride is well known to elevate blood pressure and has a variety of other negative health effects, including its contribution to increasing the risk of stroke, osteoporosis, and kidney disease. The US government has established a maximum daily intake of 2,300 milligrams (mg) of sodium, which is approximately one teaspoon; however, the majority of Americans are consuming far more.

Because sodium is naturally present in many foods, such as turkey, chicken, tomatoes, celery, kale, broccoli, and others that support essential functions within the body, there is less need for adding high amounts of salt to these and other foods. Sodium is added to foods in the grocery aisles in fairly large amounts and constitutes approximately 75 percent of the sodium consumed; read the product labels. According to the American Heart Association (AHA), any product containing the word "soda" or "sodium," for example, baking soda, monosodium glutamate, sodium nitrite, and so on, contains sodium; baking powder also contains sodium. Individual foods containing more than 480 mg of sodium and meals containing 600 mg or more are not the healthiest choices; restaurant foods can contain high amounts of sodium.

Because of the inherit health risk associated with high sodium intake and the US population's propensity to consume far more sodium than the body requires, efforts are underway by well-established and respected organizations such as the AHA to reduce the maximum daily intake of sodium to 1,500 milligrams per day. The AHA has also identified the salty six: bread and rolls, cold cuts and cured meats, pizza, poultry, soup, and fast-food sandwiches.

Finally, don't be confused over the use of sea salt as a healthy alternative to regular table salt; they both have nearly equal sodium content. Sea salt is less processed and contains a few extra minerals. Use low-sodium natural food ingredients such as onion, garlic, chives, cilantro, natural spices and herbs, and low-sodium dried seasonings (onion and garlic powder, etc.) to enhance food flavor.

Refined Sugar

Refined white sugar is commonly known as sucrose, which is made from sugar cane and sugar beets. The sugar making process includes crushing sugar cane and then refining into syrup and finally into crystals. The product is further dried, bleached, and ground into its final depleted sparkling-white form.

During the process of refining sugar, vital minerals such as calcium, potassium, magnesium, and others are removed; important vitamins such as the B complex and vitamin A are also removed. The body requires each of these elements to properly process this food substance. This devitalized food substance drains the body of important minerals and vitamins to digest, detoxify, and eliminate it. Calcium is one of the precious minerals taken from the bones to process this food substance, thereby significantly weakening the bones. White refined sugar creates a very acidic condition in the body, fueling the risk of chronic illness, such as cancer. According to www.mercola.com, refined sugar causes the bad bacteria (pathogens) in the digestive tract to grow and flourish, which greatly impacts the body's ability to absorb nutrients; essentially setting the stage for the decline of the body's overall health and function.

When this highly refined product is consumed, the B vitamin complex is seriously depleted in the cell, which contributes to a serious reduction in the production of insulin. This in turn causes a high glucose level in the blood, which can eventually create blood-vessel and cardiovascular health issues, reduce mental clarity, and threaten neurological health. Deficiency of B vitamins heightens the risk of diabetes, when the pancreas is unable to produce adequate insulin to properly control blood-sugar levels, eventually threatening the proper function and health of this critical organ.

Many health professionals also link the formation of gallstones to highly refined sugar consumption, created by high levels of improperly absorbed minerals in the blood. Sugar also makes the blood very thick and sticky, limiting much of the blood flow into small areas that supply the gums and teeth with vital nutrients and creating a variety of tooth and gum disease issues. Highly processed sugar also keeps the body hungry for nutrition and craving additional food, opening the door to several health issues, including increased risk of obesity and diabetes.

William Dufty, noted author of *Sugar Blues*, revealed in the Global Healing Center that the liver, when filled to capacity with excess sugar, releases stored glycogen (glucose) as a fatty acid into the blood where it settles in obvious areas including the breasts, belly, and buttocks, —and can eventually spill over to vital organs, creating tissue and blood issues. It's important to also note that the white blood cells can also increase and slow the body's immune system. The kidneys are working overtime to eliminate excess sugar but have to draw water from the body to accomplish this, creating thirst and a need to replenish the lost water.

Because added refined sugar in food products is not a natural or healthy source of energy and promotes weight gain, the American Heart Association (AHA) recommends that people limit intake to twenty-four grams (six teaspoons) per day for women and thirty-eight grams (nine teaspoons) for men; there are four calories in each gram of sugar. Energy from natural and healthier carbohydrate sources such as fruit, vegetables, whole grains, beans, and others is a better choice. Natural fructose in fruit should not be compared to or confused with sucrose in highly refined sugar products. The fructose in fruit combines with its natural fiber, vitamins, minerals, and phytonutrients to aid healthy brain, kidney, and other bodily functions; however, fruit should be eaten in proportion to your body requirement and health status. Conversely, *refined sugar contributes zero to health and is absolutely not required by the human body.*

Between 1970 and 2000, there was an approximate 25 percent increase of added sugar in the food supply. It's important to read food packaging nutrition labels to determine the amount of added sugar in a product. Popular brand-name iced-tea beverages contain as much as forty-eight grams of added sugar per sixteen ounces; popular and leading brands of fat-free yogurt can contain thirty grams of added sugar in a six-ounce cup. As you can see, you easily reach or exceed your added sugar limit with a serving or partial serving of your favorite food or beverage products. When you're reading labels to identify added sugar, if it ends in "ose," it's sugar! Sugar also includes syrups and masquerades as mannitol, sorbitol, xylitol, sorghum, maltodextrin, and other names.

Be careful using or avoid popular products such as agave syrup and similar sweeteners due to the high refining process used to manufacture them and their contribution to a variety of reported health issues including weight gain and heart disease. Don't be fooled by brown or raw sugar health claims; they're both refined products, with molasses added for color. Exercise caution in consuming artificial or synthetic sweeteners that are produced from chemicals; they've been linked to memory loss, tumor growth, visual disturbance, and other serious health issues. More natural sweeteners from plant sources include sucanat, stevia, and maple syrup/sugar; however, you may want to research these products and talk to your health-care provider, but exercise the same precautions concerning their use as with highly refined sugar. Honey is a natural sweetener that should be used in moderation and in accordance with your health status due to its concentrated sweetness; purchase unheated for natural vitamins and enzymes.

It's important to note that the Food and Drug Administration and the National Institute of Health classify artificial sweeteners as safe provided they're used within established limits. Research the facts and talk to your health care provider concerning their use.

A few facts concerning refined sugar (from Dr. Joseph Mercola):

- About eighteen pounds of sugar was consumed per person in 1800.
- More than half of the American population ate 180 pounds of sugar in 2009.
- In the late 1800s, there were less than three cases of diabetes per one hundred thousand people in the United States.

- Today, there are eight thousand cases of diabetes per one hundred thousand people in the United States.
- Fifteen percent of the population was obese in 1975; 32 percent of Americans today struggle with obesity.

High-Fructose Corn Syrup (HFCS)

This sweetener came on the scene in the 1960s. According to the Food and Drug Administration (FDA), the syrup is made from corn, which is converted to corn starch. Then the starch is processed into a syrup form and enzymes are added to convert some of the glucose in the syrup to fructose, resembling the composition of sucrose (table sugar). High-fructose corn syrup was chiefly developed as an alternative sweetener due to the high price of sugar and was used primarily by food and beverage manufacturers.

In the 1980s the two major soft drink producers, Coca Cola and Pepsi, began using HFCS, and early in 2000 there was as much HFCS in use as sugar. There are two basic varieties of HFCS: one used in soft drinks and a second variety used primarily in processed foods, baked goods, cereal, and other products.

Since its introduction, several health concerns have been leveled against HFCS, including the high rate of obesity, an increase in diabetes, joint inflammation, chronic liver disorders, and cardiovascular health concerns; however, the FDA has for decades classified the use of HFCS as safe. Due to the high level of negative publicity surrounding HFCS, some food and beverage manufacturers have begun to slowly return to the use of sugar in many of their products and have begun to package their products with "NO HFCS" labeling, essentially swapping one processed sugar for another.

Talk to your health-care professional if you have questions concerning the consumption of refined sugar based on your current health status.

Oils

There are several varieties of cooking and salad oils in the grocery aisles today. Popular seed, vegetable, and nut oils include canola, walnut, macadamia, soybean, corn, peanut, sunflower, cottonseed, safflower, olive, avocado, and others. Unfortunately, many of the oils, such as corn, cottonseed, grape seed, walnut, and soybean contain significantly higher ratios of inflammation-causing omega 6 polyun-saturated fatty acids with very little support and balance from omega 3 polyunsaturated fatty acids (oils contain very little omega 3); flaxseed oil is rare in containing more omega 3 than omega 6. To quiet inflamma-tion, it's important to consume foods containing omega 3 fatty acids to balance the intake of omega 6.

Healthier monounsaturated oils containing a generous amount of heart healthy omega 9 fatty acid include almond, avocado, macada-mia, olive, peanut, high oleic safflower, and sunflower oils; however, most of these oils tend to be more expensive and should be used wisely and efficiently. Cold-pressed (also known as expeller pressed), high-oleic non-GMO safflower oil is a lower cost option with one of the lowest saturated fat and highest omega 9 contents and can be used in moderate to hot-heat food preparation.

Olive oil is rich in monounsaturated fats that have actually been shown to raise HDL (good) cholesterol and lower LDL (bad) choles-terol in the bloodstream, actually contributing to heart and cardiovas-cular health. It's important to purchase pure extra virgin olive oil that has been cold-pressed and minimally processed for its antioxidant benefits. Olive oil can be used as a mixed dressing for salad and can be used in moderate-heat cooking applications.

Antioxidant-absorbing and heart-healthy extra virgin avocado oil can be used in moderate-heat cooking and also as a mixed salad oil and a drizzle on other prepared foods; macadamia nut oil is a monounsaturated oil that contains very little omega 6 fatty acid, a fair amount of antioxidants, can be used on mixed salads, and can be used in moderate-heat food preparation.

Coconut and palm oils have significantly higher saturated fat content (at 86 percent and 49 percent, respectively) than other oils; however, it's important to mention that all oils contain saturated fat, even olive oil at 14 percent and high-oleic safflower oil at 8 percent.

When selecting oils, cold-pressed oils are preferable to oils that have been extracted utilizing a very harsh heat and chemical extraction process; cold-pressed oils have a better retention of vitamin A and vitamin E antioxidants. Refined and semi-refined oils will have higher smoke points but may also contain fewer nutrients as a result of the refining process.

Although promoted as having health benefits, canola oil is a highly processed and deodorized product. Information located on Authority Nutrition's online site at authoritynutrition.com indicates that soybean and canola oils sold in the United States contain trans fat. It is highly recommended that you research and talk to your health-care provider if you have concerns related to the use of these two products. More information concerning oils can be discovered on several online sites including: http://theconsciouslife.com/omega-3-6-9-ratio-cooking-oils.htm.

It's also important to note that oil manufacturers make various health claims concerning their products. Talk to your health-care provider in making a selection that aligns with your health status and goals. Be careful to use oil in moderation and refrigerate or keep it in a cool dark place after opening; oil with rancid odor should be discarded immediately. See fried foods below in this section for more information concerning oil.

Butter

Butter is a dairy product that is produced from milk butterfat yielded primarily from cows. The milk butterfat is churned or manipulated to form a rich, sweet-tasting product that is used to top toast and bagels, flavor oatmeal and other hot cereals, and enhance the taste of an assortment of baked treats and many other cooked dishes.

Today, butter has a lot of competition from products such as margarine and other imitation butter products. Butter contains approximately eleven grams of fat per tablespoon, which includes approximately seven grams of saturated fat and three grams of monounsaturated fat. A tablespoon also contains one hundred calories, thirty milligrams of cholesterol, and no sugar.

Butter contains vitamins A, D, E, and K and important minerals, such as copper, manganese, iodine, selenium, phosphorous, and zinc. The vitamins contribute to growth and repair of cells, reducing the risk of certain cancers; calcium absorption; proper thyroid function; brain and nervous system development; and the support of healthy skin and eyes. The mineral composition supports healthy bones, healthy cell function, wound healing, and male reproduction, and provides antioxidant support. Butter contains an important phytonutrient, carotene, which provides a significant boost to the immune system and can aid in reducing the risk of some infections.

Organic butter contains natural, anti-inflammatory omega 3 fatty acid and pro-inflammatory omega 6 fatty acid; however, the omega 3 reduces the inflammatory effects of the omega 6. Essentially, butter in moderate amounts has far fewer harmful effects on the health of the cardiovascular system compared to other products, such as stick margarine or butter-type spreads; butter from pasture-fed cows is even better due to the higher quality of nutrients.

Does this mean you should start loading the popcorn with butter and putting an extra portion on your baked potato? *No.* It does mean butter contains saturated fat and should be used in moderation, especially by those attempting to reduce weight or who have other health issues that may limit or preclude its use. Be smart in consuming foods containing saturated fats; talk to your health-care professional concerning the use of this food product based on your current health status.

Margarine

Margarine was formally introduced when the French Emperor Louis Napoleon wanted to create a product to essentially replace butter for the armed forces and people with lower economic means. Margarine has undergone significant updates and changes since its introduction approximately 145 years ago, including color, ingredients, and manufacturing processes; many consumer and health advocate demands have brought attention to this product.

Today, margarine is a vegetable-based food that undergoes significant chemical manipulation and processing to resemble butter. The oil from the plant used in margarine (corn, safflower, etc.) is subjected to the hydrogenation process, which essentially infuses hydrogen into the oil via a high temperature and pressure method, making the oil solid and similar to the look of butter. As a result of the hydrogenation process, trans–fatty acids (trans fats) are created. Today, trans fats are the greatest health concern among the various forms of fats—more so than saturated fats.

The major health issues associated with trans fats is the tremendous stress placed on the body to metabolize or process it, its contribution to inflammation, and its ability to increase LDL (bad) cholesterol and decrease HDL (good) cholesterol, which significantly increases the risk of coronary heart disease as a result of plaque buildup in the arteries. Margarine in stick or block form contains a higher amount of trans fats than the soft tub spreads and blends being created today as a result of the health community's expressed concerns. However, manufacturers can indicate the tub product contains no trans fats if it has less than 0.5 percent trans fat (that's still trans fat).

Read the label. If it contains hydrogenated, partially hydrogenated, shortening, or glycerides, put the product back on the shelf and search the aisles for something healthier; you owe that to yourself. It's amazing that science has been tinkering with this food product for nearly a century and a half and still seems unable to fully satisfy the various public suspicions and concerns. Because trans fat is unnatural, eating whole foods limits their use and resolves much of the concern. Talk to your health-care professional if you have concerns or questions related to this food.

Fried Foods

Let me start by saying, I'm only the messenger. Foods lose many of their vitamins and minerals when fried. When something is fried in oil, it can also double or triple the calories. A large baked potato contains 220 calories and 0.2 grams of fat. A fitday.com research article related to food myths reveals that when the same potato is sliced and fried, it contains nearly 700 calories and 34 grams of fat—seriously. Regular fried-food consumption can also contribute to major health challenges, including significant cardiovascular issues. There is also an increased risk of colon, lung, breast, prostate and other cancers caused by carcinogenic compounds that can surface when animal or plant foods are fried at high temperatures. As mentioned earlier, the Mayo Clinic's research has discovered that regularly eating a single serving of fried fish per week increases the risk of heart failure by 50 percent; think about it!

The information also reports that some restaurants use less expensive partially hydrogenated oils, which contain high levels of trans fats that pose very serious health issues. It's well known that these health concerns include the increase of LDL (bad) cholesterol and decrease of HDL (good) cholesterol, significantly contributing to heart disease and stroke.

Reuse of oil and frying beyond the smoke point poses a health risk due to continual oxidation of the oil, which creates further challenges for the body. When the oil decomposes it produces carcinogenic compounds; decomposition is noticeable when vapor is released from the oil. Eating foods cooked in decomposed oil is very threatening to your health; inhaling the oil vapor should also be avoided.

If you insist on frying, almond, avocado, and macadamia oils have moderate smoke points and contain very little omega 6 polyunsaturated fatty acid; however, they're expensive oil products. Non-GMO cold-pressed, high-oleic safflower oil is lower cost monounsaturated oil with a slightly higher smoke point, adding better protection from oil decomposition. Talk to your health-care provider in making an oil selection that aligns with your health status and goals. Be careful to use oil in moderation.

Be smart in your food choices and food preparation. Oven baking or "fake fried" may be an alternative to frying. Oven baked "fake fries" or baked chicken properly seasoned and coated with whole-grain, unbleached, and unbromated flour (set for a few minutes to allow some of the flour to absorb) and baked with moderate heat to an internal temperature of 165 degrees Fahrenheit provides a flavorful golden and crispy texture; research alternative baking or sautéing for the foods you're currently frying. Remove the skin from poultry and fish before consuming. Talk to your health-care professional concerning the risk of fried foods.

Phytic Acid (Phytates)

Phytic acid, commonly referred to as phytates, is the main storage form of phosphorous found in grains, nuts, seeds, and beans; phosphorous is required for the germination and growth of the plant. The phytates protect the plant during its maturing process from various damaging environmental challenges.

A compelling issue associated with phytates is that they're not digestible by humans and bind to important minerals such as calcium, magnesium, iron, and zinc, preventing their absorption, which is why phytates are often referred to as antinutrients. Phytates also interfere with important enzymes required to digest food. Humans lack a sufficient level of the enzyme phytase to properly break down and absorb phytic acid.

The amount of phytic acid varies among grains, nuts, seeds, and beans; a high level of phytates resides in the coating of bran-based foods such as rice bran and wheat bran. According to the Weston A. Price Foundation's online site at www.westonaprice.org, Brazil nuts, brown rice, almonds, walnuts, and cocoa powder contain some of the highest levels of phytic acid.

Our ancestors and different cultures from around the world routinely prepared grains, nuts, seeds, and beans utilizing various soaking, grinding, and fermentation methods prior to eating them. Modern and faster living today has pushed most of these preparations aside in favor of more immediate routines of consumption. Improved calcium absorption and minimization of premature bone loss is just one example of what can occur when phytic acid is reduced. Other health benefits of phytic acid reduction include increased production of enzymes and increased strength of vital nutrients, such as vitamin B and others. Eating vinegar-based food products and foods rich in vitamin C with foods containing phytic acid may offset some of the antinutrient activity.

Visit www.westonaprice.org/health-topics/living-with-phytic-acid/ or other online websites for additional information concerning phytic acid and proper food preparation. For those interested in speeding phytic acid removal who may not read the available information at westonaprice.org, add an acid such as lemon or vinegar to the soaking water for beans and grain such as brown rice. Soak rice for twelve to twenty-four hours and beans for twenty-four to forty-eight hours, changing the water once or twice and adding acid each time; soaking also helps to reduce gas in the beans. For nuts, add a teaspoon of salt to the soaking water to improve enzyme activity and soak for twelve to eighteen hours, changing the water once or twice and adding salt each time. You can dry nuts in the oven at a low temperature of 175 degrees Fahrenheit for approximately three hours until nuts are sufficiently dried for consumption. You can soak the aforementioned foods for less time to at least remove some of the phytic acid.

Fasting

This is a very personal decision with benefits. The most basic benefit is that you give your body an opportunity to rest from the rigors of eating, digesting, absorbing, and eliminating. We voluntarily fast during religious time frames such as the Lenten season and during other observances. We naturally fast during periods of sleep, and the body knows to automatically fast during periods of illness.

Consistent overeating is a true enemy to longevity and one of the most dangerous things anyone can do to the body. Conversely, taking an intermittent or longer break can do wonders in rejuvenating the body and oftentimes restore vitality to important functions within the body. If you're a reasonably smart person, you know when it's time to slow down and take a break; your body will provide the necessary prompts. It's important to stay properly hydrated during your fasting break. Talk to your health-care professional concerning fasting and other decisions that may impact your health status.

It's important to remember the spiritual aspects of fasting and its powerful ability to create an unbreakable bond with our Father. Recall Jesus, who transcended worldly temptation in his journey to glory and eternity when he elected to fast for forty days. Matthew, chapter 6, teaches us "When you fast, do not look somber as the hypocrites do… so that it will not be obvious to men that you are fasting, but only to your Father, who is unseen…."

Food for Thought

- Soak beans, nuts and seeds, and grains (brown rice) to reduce and/or remove the antinutrient phytic acid (see phytic acid above in this section).
- Read food package labels to detect added sodium and sugar.

- Added refined white sugar adds zero to health and is absolutely not required by the human body.
- Balance omega 6 with omega 3 fatty acid to quiet inflammation.
- Olive oil is rich in monounsaturated fats and has actually been shown to raise HDL (good) cholesterol and lower LDL (bad) cholesterol in the bloodstream.
- All oils contain saturated fat, even olive oil at 14 percent and high-oleic safflower oil at 8 percent.
- Limit saturated fat to 10 percent or less of daily calories; eat butter sparingly.
- *Avoid* trans-fat foods such as stick margarine completely. Eat more whole food instead of this unnatural and unhealthy man-made substance lingering in hydrogenated food products.
- A potato containing 220 calories and less than one gram of fat increases to 700 calories and 34 grams of fat when sliced and fried—just the messenger.
- Bake instead of frying; you may live longer and healthier.
- If health status permits and with your health-care provider's awareness, a brief fasting break from eating, digesting, absorbing, and eliminating food can actually be beneficial and rejuvenating; stay properly hydrated during this time.

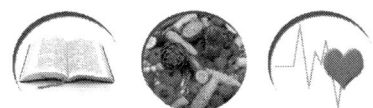

CHAPTER 12

WHAT IS THIS STUFF? (FOOD ADDITIVES)

Ever wonder what some of those fifteen ingredients in the foods you purchase really are and how they impact your health? Time and space don't permit a close examination of the thousands of food additives, but they do provide an opportunity to discuss some of the issues associated with food additives and a further opportunity to encourage you to read labels and to begin to research these synthetic materials before you consume them. It's similar to when we were kids and our parents would tell us not to put certain things in our mouth because they knew the risk and harm associated with doing so. It's the same thing with some of these additives. This passage is not intended to scare anyone, but to educate individuals on the importance of understanding what they're consuming.

Ruth Winter is the author of a 579-page book entitled *A Consumer's Dictionary of Food Additives*, in which she identifies over *twelve thousand* food additives, many of which have very mysterious and scientific names, and various impacts on our health. In her book, Ms. Winter categorizes food additives as preservatives, neutralizers, humectants, ripeners, bleaching and maturing agents, processing aids, texturizers or stabilizers, coloring agents, flavorings, nutrition supplements, and miscellaneous additives.

Writers of The Mindful Word at mindfulword.org remind us that the fact that an additive is approved by a regulating entity doesn't make it safe. There are food additives currently in use that pose a range of questions related to their safety. Food experts and writers cite examples of food additives that were once classified as safe for consumption; however, products containing these additives had to be removed from the grocery shelf because they were later discovered to have serious and damaging health impacts. Questionable food additives are often disguised and hide behind other names; for example, MSG, an excitotoxin (flavor enhancer) heavily linked to obesity and neurologic health issues, including headaches, assumes other names such as hydrolyzed vegetable protein, whey protein, autolyzed yeast, yeast extract, or natural flavors—ever wonder why some restaurant foods are so highly seasoned and tasty?

Some current food additives have been associated with chronic diseases, such as asthma and cancer. Other serious health issues associated with additives include memory loss, visual disturbance, migraines, skin disorders, hyperactivity in children, and a host of other major health issues. It's important for you, the consumer, to research these additives. Why would you not be concerned about fifteen different chemical ingredients that you can barely pronounce being in your food? Eat whole foods or foods with fewer ingredients. Purchasing foods that contain a myriad of ingredients, particularly ingredients that are completely foreign and raise specific questions related to their purpose, may not be the better choice until some level of research has been completed. If a product contains that many strange ingredients, put it back on the shelf!

Do your research to discover what things like propylene glycol monoesters and soy lecithin in cake and cookie mixes really are. What exactly are cellulose and xanthan gums in bakery products used for, and how do they impact your specific health? Ever wonder what BHA & BHT, sodium nitrate, aspartame, parabens, and sulfites mean to your health after consuming them from a variety of products? You owe it to yourself to determine what these food additives really are and how they impact your health. Check out this article at Mindful Momma's online site concerning a few of the additives: http://mindfulmomma. com/2015/01/the-12-worst-food-additives-and-where-youll-find-them.html. Talk to your health-care provider if you have questions or concerns.

Food for Thought:

- If a product has a high number of ingredients you either can't pronounce or are totally unfamiliar with, put it back on the shelf and go find a better food.
- Food additive names are often disguised as something else; be careful.
- The fact that a regulating entity says it's safe doesn't make it safe; do your research and talk to your health-care provider if you have concerns.
- Eat more whole foods and less processed food with multiple artificial additives; your body will likely thank you by getting healthier.

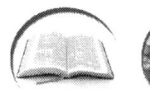 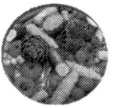 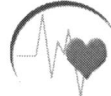

CHAPTER 13

A FEW IMPORTANT TERMS

Whole Foods: Foods that are in their natural, unprocessed state, many of which have been discussed in detail earlier in this book, including fruits, vegetables, whole grains, nuts, seeds, beans, poultry, and fish. Foods in a raw or necessary prepared form with very little to no substantive change. Foods that have the capacity to heal and the ability to provide the body with the essential vitamins, minerals, fiber, and phytonutrients required for sustainable health. Other definitions of whole foods include foods that are not processed or refined and contain no additives such as salt, sugar, fat, or any other added ingredients.

Organic Food: This term primarily refers to how the foods in this group were grown. Organic refers to the organic farming practices that cultivate and enrich the land and soil where foods are produced, guided by strict organic farming standards. Essentially, organic food has to be produced without the use of engineered seeds and chemically based pesticides and fertilizers. Organic refers not only to plants grown under organic guidelines, but it also refers to dairy and animal products that are provided from animals who consume organic feed to produce meat, poultry, yogurt, eggs, and other products; animals producing organic products are not fed any antibiotics or growth hormones. Organic foods also include packaged food products that were created with organic based ingredients, for example, bread, dairy, snack foods, and others.

It's important to note that some organically grown food products, such as tomatoes, blueberries, strawberries, and other berries, actually have higher nutritional value, particularly antioxidant strength, than conventionally grown tomatoes and berries; however, this doesn't apply to all organically grown foods. Ongoing research is being conducted to determine whether greater health benefits are present in other organically grown foods.

Organic foods are classified based on the amount of organic ingredients contained in the food. As you might expect, whole foods such as fruits and vegetables that are grown organically are classified as 100 percent organic; other foods containing only organic ingredients can also be classified as 100 percent organic. Foods that contain at least 95 percent organic ingredients are labeled "organic"; foods with 70–95 percent organic ingredients are identified as "containing organic ingredients"; and foods containing less than 70 percent organic ingredients can only list the organic ingredients in the food label.

Genetically Modified Organism (GMO): The World Health Organization describes genetically modified organisms (GMOs) as "organisms (plants, animals, or microorganisms) in which the genetic material (DNA) has been altered in a way that does not occur naturally by mating and/or natural recombination." This phenomenon is also known as genetic engineering—essentially placing DNA from one organism into another organism. Foods today can be genetically engineered for a variety of reasons, including increasing crop yield for global feeding, decreasing production cost, improving drought resistance, and creating stronger, disease-resistant crops. According to the Non-GMO Project, in 2009, 93 percent of soy and 86 percent of corn were GMOs. It's estimated that 90 percent of crops grown for canola are GMOs.

There are many public concerns and questions related to GMO foods, including their consumption safety. Unfortunately, there are not a lot of answers to many of these questions and concerns; however, the increased demand to have stores label non-GMO products is showing significant results. Check with your local grocery stores to see what they're doing to provide education and responses to any concerns you may have.

Cholesterol: A waxy fat substance in the blood produced by the liver and also obtained from animal food sources. It has a variety of important functions, including building and maintaining healthy cells; manufacturing specific hormones; and aiding the liver in producing bile, which is critical to the digestion of fat in food. Because of its inability to travel in our water-based blood, cholesterol is carried in the blood via an enclosed vessel called a lipoprotein. A blood test is the standard way to measure and determine blood cholesterol levels and issues.

Cholesterol is separated into two basic categories that combine to give you a total count: low density lipoprotein (LDL/bad) cholesterol that potentially clogs the arteries and contributes to an increased risk of heart disease and stroke, and high density lipoprotein (HDL/good) cholesterol that acts as a cleaning solution to prevent cholesterol buildup in the arteries. According to the American Heart Association, desirable LDL cholesterol would be 100 mg/dl or less, and desirable HDL cholesterol would be above 60 mg/dl; a total cholesterol number significantly less than 200 is desirable. Triglyceride is a fat in the blood and is the third leg of the stool that can also create cardiovascular issues and is also transported via the lipoprotein vessel; less than 150 mg/dl is desirable.

Eating fresh fruits and vegetables, especially those rich in soluble fiber like apples, oranges, berries, carrots, sweet potatoes, and cucumbers; whole grains, especially oats, including oatmeal and low-sugar, whole-oat cereals; walnuts; and black beans, together with reducing saturated and trans fats, staying physically active, and reducing excess weight are key factors in lowering LDL and increasing HDL blood cholesterol levels. Monounsaturated and polyunsaturated fat, regarded as good fat, are known to aid the lowering of LDL and increase HDL cholesterol (see fats under macronutrients section). Cholesterol is not found in many plant foods; it's found primarily in meat, eggs, cheese, and shrimp. Talk to your health-care provider about questions you may have concerning cholesterol.

Probiotics: Live bacteria which enhances and supports the good bacteria in the body.   The approved scientific definition developed by the Food and Agricultural Organization of the UN and the World Health Organization describes probiotics as "live microorganisms that, when administered in adequate amounts, confer a health benefit on the host." The science community is very strict in defining probiotics as having identifiable and specific health benefits. Research information on the Live Science online site at www.livescience.com indicates that yogurt, with its standard bacteria, is considered a probiotic because it helps lactose-intolerant individuals digest the yogurt; however, the standard bacteria does not survive the travel through the entire digestive tract. The information points out that added bacteria in yogurt (lactobacilli and bifidobacteria) in addition to the yogurt cultures, can survive the voyage all the way into the colon. The added bacteria join and support the good bacteria already residing in the colon, increasing the bacterial health of the digestive tract. Check the yogurt ingredient label for added bacteria.

Macrobiotics: A holistic approach to human health and healing that includes a diet of whole cereal grains, vegetables, soups, beans, and sea vegetables.

Enzymes: Protein molecules made by amino acids and strategically located in specific areas of the body. Each specific enzyme has a particular function and that function only. As part of the transformation activity, enzymes act as a catalyst to facilitate a required change or transformation, for example, transforming starch to glucose to be used for energy. Enzymes are not part of the changed substance; they only act as the change agent and can be reused for their specific purpose. Some people may lack a particular enzyme for a specific function, for example, the lactase enzyme to break down milk sugar, or lactose, thereby creating a condition of lactose intolerance. According to Healing Daily at www.healingdaily.com and other science studies, enzymes in raw or whole food digest faster and easier than those in cooked foods. Many health scientists argue that cooking food can damage food enzymes and weakens their nutritional impact; however, several foods require some form of cooking for proper digestion.

Metabolism: The chemical processes that occur in the body's cells to generate or transfer energy to facilitate the *speed* of all bodily functions, including digestion, waste elimination, blood circulation, proper brain/muscle/and nerve function, respiration, body temperature, and all other functions. In short, metabolism is the process that involves your body transforming what you consume into energy. Your body requires energy even when you're at rest, so that the aforementioned bodily functions can continue. Exercise is well known to boost a sluggish metabolism; stay hydrated to maintain a healthy metabolism.

Metabolic Syndrome: A grouping of specific medical conditions, including low levels of HDL (good) cholesterol, high levels of blood sugar, high triglycerides (fat) levels in the blood, high blood pressure, and excess weight around the midsection, all of which place you in a high-risk category for heart disease, stroke, and diabetes; these groups are indicators that something is not occurring as designed. This diagnosis occurs when a person has at least three of the risk factors. According to Dr. John A. McDougall in the McDougall Newsletter, many researchers consider insulin resistance to be a key factor in the cause of metabolic syndrome. Consult with your health-care professional for proper treatment concerning these and other risk factors.

Electrolytes: Composed of minerals in the body's blood supply, which contain an electrical charge for regulating blood pressure, cell integrity, and proper muscle and nerve function and maintaining fluid levels, blood pH (alkaline and acid balance), energy levels, brain function, heartbeat, and other critical bodily functions. Potassium, sodium, magnesium, chloride, calcium, and phosphorous are the common electrolytes in the body and are needed in certain combinations to conduct these specific bodily functions. Electrolytes are controlled by various hormones in the body, which are created primarily by the kidneys and adrenal glands. Proper hydration is important in maintaining electrolyte balance; imbalance can create serious health issues and bodily dysfunction. Be careful of added sugar content and other ingredients in beverages containing chemically added electrolytes; for better health, eat balanced meals containing the electrolyte minerals mentioned above.

pH (Power of Hydrogen): The basic pH scale and range is 0 to 14. The pH of water is 7.0, and the acid-base balance for human blood ranges from 7.35 to 7.45; 7.4 is considered ideal. A blood pH higher than 7.0 would be considered alkaline (oxygen-rich) and lower than 7.0 would be registered as acidic (oxygen-poor); pH levels in other areas of the body, such as the digestive tract, vary from the blood pH.

An overly acidic body decreases cellular function and is a great environment for debilitating and chronic diseases such as cancer, arthritis, asthma, immune dysfunction, heart disease, acid reflux, and others; the body does not properly absorb healing nutrients in an acidic state. Acid-producing foods include alcohol, meat, dairy, nuts, corn, wheat, and refined sugars. Fruits and vegetables, particularly those containing sufficient amounts of potassium, reduce acidic conditions in the body and reduce the strain on the body's acid-reducing systems; decreasing salt intake and staying hydrated are also helpful. Lemon has an alkalizing effect in the body and is considered one of the best alkalizing agents; apples, cucumbers, grapes, carrots, collard greens, kale, romaine lettuce, avocados, bananas, strawberries, broccoli, sweet potatoes, bell peppers, green beans, and a host of other fruits and vegetables are great alkalizing agents as well.

Circadian Rhythm: The body's natural twenty-four-hour rhythm is governed by the cellular biological clocks located throughout the body, all of which are controlled and coordinated by the master clock located in the brain. This around-the-clock rhythm influences respiration, blood pressure, body temperature, and other critical functions.

This natural rhythm is disrupted and a significant burden is placed on the body by filling it with foods, such as saturated fats, that cause the body to utilize greater energy as a result of the extended periods of digestion and processing that are created by such foods. This takes precious time away from rejuvenation and healing, further disrupting the natural body rhythms. Disruption can also occur if eating occurs during the latest hours of the day. If unavoidable, select easily digestible food so that the body is able to process the final meal with as little energy as possible in order to maintain its natural rhythm of absorbing nutrients and preparing for rest. The body should not be in a heavy digestion and processing state in the late evening; the body is rejuvenated and heals much better when resting soundly.

Important Rhythm Approximations (blissreturned.wordpress.com):

- Deepest sleep occurs at approximately 2:00 a.m.
- The greatest rise in blood pressure occurs at approximately 6:45 a.m.
- Highest level of alertness occurs at approximately 10:00 a.m.
- Highest blood pressure occurs at approximately 6:30 p.m.

Food for Thought:

- Even a basic understanding of important body chemistry and functions as they relate to your well-being is important; knowledge is power.
- Many researchers consider insulin resistance to be a key factor in the cause of metabolic syndrome.
- Be careful of added sugar content and other ingredients in beverages containing chemically added electrolytes.
- Eat alkaline foods and limit acid-causing foods; chronic illness loves an acidic body.
- Added bacteria in yogurt (lactobacilli and bifidobacteria) in addition to the yogurt cultures, can survive the voyage all the way into the colon thereby increasing the bacterial health of the digestive tract.
- Cholesterol is found primarily in nonplant foods, including meat, eggs, cheese, and shrimp; total cholesterol should be less than 200.
- Eat more whole natural foods as opposed to processed foods for sustainable health; choose organic when possible.
- Eat healthy foods, drink water, and rest at proper times; for better sleep, refrain from eating meals late in the evening.

- Many health scientists argue that cooking food can damage food enzymes and weaken their nutritional impact; however, several foods require some form of cooking for proper digestion.
- Some organic food products, such as tomatoes, blueberries, strawberries, and other berries, actually have higher nutritional value, particularly antioxidant strength, than conventionally grown tomatoes or berries; however, this doesn't apply to all organically grown foods.

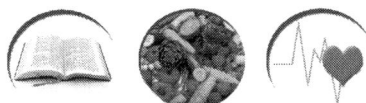

CHAPTER 14

IF BODY PARTS COULD TALK (LET'S LISTEN)

"Do not be wise in your own eyes; fear the Lord and shun evil. This will bring health to your body and nourishment to your bones."
—PROVERBS 3:7–8 (NIV)

Heart: I am a muscle located in the center of your chest with a slight tilt to the left. My main purpose is to pump oxygen-filled blood to all the organs and tissues throughout the body via the blood circulatory system. The circulatory system sends blood from me to the lungs where it picks up oxygen and sends the oxygenated blood back to me where I then pump it out to the tissues via the arteries. The blood will return to me to repeat the cycle; the continual pumping is my heartbeat. My level of work depends on the demands you place upon me; for example, exercise, digestion of unhealthy foods, stress, strenuous work or activity, excessive weight, and other demands cause me to work harder. I can beat well over one hundred thousand times daily depending on the demand.

An assortment of foods containing vitamins, minerals, phytonutrients, and fiber contribute to my overall health. Potassium-rich foods, such as bananas and avocados, help reduce the pressure inside the blood I am pumping, which relaxes the blood vessels and stimulates increased blood flow for me to operate more effectively; reducing salt is critical and improves my performance. I also enjoy foods such as to-matoes, blueberries, grapes, oranges, watermelon, broccoli, bell pep-pers, beans, peas, oatmeal, omega 3–rich fish such as salmon, and other foods that contribute to my health and strength. Please don't let me forget to ask you to drink plenty of fresh water and to stop smoking.

The Center for Disease Control and Prevention indicates that Americans suffer over 1.5 million heart attacks and strokes annually, and nearly 44 percent of African American men and 48 percent of African American women have some form of cardiovascular disease. The American Heart Association reports that heart disease and stroke are the leading causes of death of women in the United States and kill nearly fifty thousand African American women annually.

Brain: I'm a very important part of the human body located beneath the skull. I am made up of 75 percent water and have the responsibil-ity of operating as the central command office for the nervous system. I work very closely with the spinal cord and sensory components—touch, vision, sound, and so on—to accomplish much of my work. I also regulate involuntary functions such as breathing and digestion.

My left side controls the muscles on the right and my right side controls the muscle activity on the left. My left side is generally associ-ated with motor skills involving speech, recall of information, problem solving, and language. The right tends to be my more creative side. I utilize approximately one-fifth of all oxygen and blood circulating in the body and 25 percent of glucose energy. Antioxidants and healthy whole foods such as blueberries and strawberries, dark green leafy vegetables, broccoli, carrots, sweet potatoes, omega 3 fatty fish such as salmon and sardines, walnuts, and others are great nourishment for me. Staying active and getting exercise that utilizes clean, fresh air is also important for my well-being; fresh water is critically important for my proper hydration and clarity. Dangerous and toxic metals, including aluminum, tend to settle in my tissue, contributing to neurodegenerative disorders such as Alzheimer's disease; read product labels to avoid products containing any form of toxic ingredients such as aluminum (see the next chapter, "More Tips and Tidbits").

Liver: I'm the largest internal organ in the body, designed to work as a filter in your digestive system. I'm a storage facility for energy, can regulate blood sugar, and make enzymes, among other things. Everything you eat and drink has to pass through me for reassembly into something useful the body requires for building and maintaining overall health. To protect your cells and tissues from damage, I convert fat-soluble toxic materials into water-soluble materials for easier elimination. No matter how much insult and abuse you hurl at me by eating and drinking unhealthy foods and beverages, such as greasy potato chips and fried foods, fat-filled meat, sugary/corn syrup or alcohol-filled beverages, and excessive sodium in packaged food, I remain loyal in performing my job to filter and process these harmful elements into something useful and separate and filter out the toxic poisons for elimination from the body.

Constant abuse will eventually slow me down and one day renders me ineffective to support you. Fatty liver disease, cirrhosis, inflammation, and swelling are many of my abused conditions and can lead to the development of arthritis, diabetes, high blood pressure, and other health issues for you. Heavy use of over-the-counter drugs such as acetaminophen can contribute to my premature failure. However, I operate best and can sometimes heal myself when you send me fresh, whole foods such as fruits, vegetables, seeds and nuts, and whole grains that I can easily convert into the nutrients you need to keep your engines running smoothly. Water, lemons, apples, carrots and juice, sweet potatoes, red bell peppers, green leafy vegetables, walnuts, broccoli, garlic, beets, lentils, avocados, pumpkin seeds, and others are some of my best friends for detoxification.

Lungs: I'm a major part of the body's respiratory system. I'm located on the left and right sides of the chest, and am responsible for providing oxygen to the blood; our neighbor, the heart, lives between us. I am filled with multiple air passageways creating the respiratory tract, which receives fresh air for the purpose of generating the precious oxygen your tissues and organs require. I expand to let fresh air in as you inhale and return to size when you exhale to let air out. I receive blood with very little oxygen from my neighbor, the heart, and I refill it with oxygen and return the oxygenated blood to the heart via the pulmonary vein, so the heart can do its job of pumping it to the various tissue stations; I simultaneously exhale the carbon dioxide gas that's brought back to me. My friend the brain controls my rate of breathing and sends the required messages to speed up my breathing if carbon dioxide gas collects in excess and needs to be exhaled.

Fresh water, fruits, vegetables, nuts, beans, and other fresh, whole foods with their wide array of vitamins, minerals, and phytonutrients are what I enjoy the most. I'm at my best when you provide foods that sustain and improve my health, including red bell peppers with their vitamin C and phytonutrients; oranges with their rich supply of vitamin C and B vitamins; my good friend the apple, which is showing signs of protecting me from cancer; pomegranate for reducing tumor growth; carrots and sweet potatoes for their rich vitamin A and C and phytonutrient content that reduces the risk of lung disease; the infection-fighting power of onions; broccoli and kale with their chlorophyll content that has demonstrated results of reducing the risk of lung cancer; beans and nuts with their rich supply of magnesium; and many other foods are helpful as well. Please avoid fried foods and eliminate the use of tobacco for my good health. The National Cancer Institute indicates that more people in the United States die from lung cancer than any other form of cancer.

According to the United States Department of Health and Human Services Office of Minority Health, African Americans are 20 percent more likely to develop asthma than whites, and 2.8 million African Americans reported having asthma in 2012. African American children are three times more likely to be admitted to the hospital for asthma compared to white children and had a death rate seven times that of white children in 2003–2005; secondhand tobacco exposure is an identified contributor to this respiratory disease for minority children.

Kidneys: There are two of us whose main function is to filter the blood; all blood passes through us multiple times each day to remove toxic waste. We regulate fluid and electrolyte balance and create urine, which is eliminated from the bladder, as part of our filtering duties. We also regulate the levels of potassium, acid, and salt in the body and produce hormones that affect blood pressure and the production of red blood cells. Foods that we enjoy that provide valuable nutrients for our health and well-being include fresh water, red grapes, red bell peppers, blueberries, strawberries, cherries, apples, cabbage, onions, garlic, olive oil, and other whole foods that reduce the risk of chronic and inflammatory disease in support of renal health. We're not big on refined white sugar.

Some of the frequent issues we face are chronic kidney disease such as diabetes as well as kidney stones and urinary tract infections. It's important to note that diabetes can lead to heart attack and stroke and is a major contributor to nerve damage and vision impairment, including blindness. Diabetes can also damage us and lead to kidney failure; high blood pressure can create complications for us as well. According to the online site www.livestrong.com, weakened kidney conditions reduce filtering capacity and call for a reduction in foods with high phosphorous, potassium, and sodium content; protein should also be reduced to minimize accumulation of acidic waste. Talk to your health-care provider concerning proper foods to eat or avoid in maintaining healthy blood-sugar levels and sustaining kidney health.

According to the United States Department of Health and Human Services Office of Minority Health, African Americans are 80 percent more likely to be diagnosed with diabetes than whites and twice as likely to die from complications of diabetes as whites. It is critically important to control blood-sugar levels; blood sugar less than 120 is good, but less than 100 is ideal.

Pancreas: I'm a single organ located in the abdomen behind the stomach and vital to digestion and regulating blood-sugar levels. I produce insulin when necessary to counteract high levels of sugar entering the blood, which are often created by high levels of refined carbohydrates entering the digestive system. I also make enzymes to digest fats, carbohydrates, and proteins in the intestine and create the necessary enzymes to aid digestion. I help my neighbor, the liver, store glucose, and I am instrumental in ensuring muscle and tissue use glucose properly for energy. I also produce the hormone glucagon, which contributes to balancing blood sugar by raising it when necessary; glucagon's function is opposite that of insulin.

Some of the conditions that affect me are pancreatitis (inflammation), pancreatic cancer, and diabetes. Some of the nourishing foods I enjoy are blueberries, cherries, sweet potatoes, spinach, broccoli, and garlic, all containing healing and health-sustaining antioxidant phytonutrients, vitamins, and minerals that reduce the risk of several chronic and inflammatory diseases, including the cell-damaging effects of cancer. I also enjoy better health if you limit the amount of red meat and processed foods you consume.

Breasts: The breasts of a woman generally begin growth and development at puberty; generally between nine and twelve years of age. The breasts are composed of fatty tissue and contain multiple mammary glands that are able to produce milk. One of the most insidious and challenging health issues today for women is breast cancer. According to Susan G. Komen, breast cancer occurs when cells in the breast divide and grow without normal control; more than half of breast cancer begins in the milk ducts. Cancers in other parts of the body can move and metastasize in the breasts. Over 230,000 new cases of invasive breast cancer and over 40,000 breast-cancer deaths will occur in the United States in 2015. Self-exams and regular screenings are highly recommended!

According to the Black Women's Health Imperative (BWHI), black women are less likely to get breast cancer throughout their lifespan, but have a higher rate of death when it's contracted. Breast cancer is the leading cancer death among black women ages forty-five to sixty-four, and according to a Center for Disease Control study, African American women deaths in that age bracket were 60 percent higher than white women. Younger black women up to age forty-four have a higher incidence of breast cancer; aggressive forms of breast cancer appear in younger black women. According to BWHI, black women have denser breast tissue, which make small growths harder to detect; however, regular screening before growths are evident is critically important. For more information, visit the Black Women's Health Imperative online at www.bwhi.org/issues-and-resources/black-women-and-breast-cancer/.

Also, the *Journal of Clinical Oncology* article "Insulin Breast Cancer Connection: Confirmatory Data Set the Stage for Better Care" at http://jco.ascopubs.org/content/ 29/1/7.full states that high insulin levels and type 2 diabetes have a strong correlation to breast-cancer development. Ladies, it is critically important to maintain a healthy weight and to limit or avoid eating unhealthy processed foods that continually increase blood sugar and insulin levels. It's also important to limit or avoid the consumption of high fat foods such as meat, fried foods, and high-fat dairy because of their ability to increase estrogen production, which contributes to an increased risk of cancer growth in the breast; estrogen is produced in fat tissue. The American Cancer Society also recommends limiting the use of alcohol to decrease the risk of breast cancer.

Proper nutrition plays an enormous role in maintaining overall health and in reducing the risk of disease, including breast cancer; fresh air, exercise, plenty of water, fresh fruits and vegetables, and other healthy foods are an important component of reducing the risk. According to Everyday Health's online site at www.everyday-health.com, some of the more nutritious foods include broccoli, collard greens, kale, brussels sprouts, and cabbage for blocking tumor growth and tumor migration (travel); apples for their fiber and phytonutrient compounds; pomegranate for its cancer-fighting phytonutrients; walnuts' omega 3 fatty acids for slowing the growth of tumors (eat sparingly); wild-caught omega 3 fatty fish, such as salmon, mackerel, and tuna; foods containing carotenoids such as oranges, carrots, cantaloupe, peaches/nectarines, and sweet pota-toes; high-antioxidant berries, including blueberries, strawberries, blackberries, and raspberries; garlic; and green tea, which has dem-onstrated the ability to reduce tumor growth. These are but a few of the foods that have shown beneficial health effects that can support breast health.

Prostate: I'm a small gland about the size of a walnut located below the bladder, part of the male reproductive system. The prostate is instrumental in providing and adding prostatic fluid to seminal fluid as part of the process that creates semen and also aids in channeling the semen; sperm travels in the semen. Currently, a prostate-specific antigen (PSA) blood exam combined with the digital rectal exam is the widely used method to determine prostate health; I know fellas, I know (put your big man shoes on)!

The prostate increases in size as a man ages and can crowd the urethra, which can cause issues related to the proper release of urine. The enlarged prostate is referred to as benign prostatic hyperplasia (BPH) and is common in men age sixty and can affect 90 percent of men age seventy and older. According to the American Cancer Society, approximately 190,000 men are diagnosed with prostate cancer each year. African American men are far more likely to contract the disease and twice as likely as white men to die from the disease. Men should have regular health screenings, especially if they have first degree (direct) family members who have experienced prostate disease. Dr. Isaac Powell, professor of urology at Wayne State University School of Medicine and Karmanos Cancer Institute, believes African American men should begin screening at age thirty-five to decrease the mortality-rate disparity.

To reduce the risk of prostate cancer, it's important to eat fresh fruits and vegetables, especially those rich in the phytonutrient lycopene, including tomatoes and tomato products, watermelon, papaya, and pink grapefruit. Pomegranate, strawberries, blackberries, raspberries, walnuts, black beans, kale, broccoli, cabbage, and cauliflower also support prostate health. Garlic, onions, mushrooms, and sunflower seeds are foods rich in selenium, the antioxidant support mineral that is known to have beneficial effects on prostate health. Men should also limit or avoid the consumption of red meat and processed red meat products, fried foods, and high-fat dairy to reduce prostate cancer risks. Excessive calcium intake can also negatively affect prostate health. Men, talk to your health-care provider prior to taking high doses of vitamin E and selenium supplements due to a possible increase in prostate-cancer risk (see omega 3 under Fats for other prostate health information).

The 100 Black Men of Greater Detroit and Blue Cross Blue Shield of Michigan are leading the fight and encouraging men in the metropolitan Detroit area to get screened through their "Man Up" efforts!

Esophagus: I'm the approximately eight-to-ten-inch tube that connects the throat and stomach. My walls contract to move food into the stomach for digestion, and my lining is filled with glands to keep my passageway moist so that I can allow easier movement of food. Some of the health conditions that affect me are esophageal cancer, heartburn, gastroesophageal reflux disease (GERD), and other conditions. Certain medications for blood pressure, asthma, depression, and other conditions or issues may increase the risk of reflux disease; smoking, alcohol, and caffeine consumption may also aggravate the disease. An upper endoscopy is a common exam that reviews the condition of the esophagus, stomach, and small intestines. According to Dr. Mark Hyman, a sustainable solution may also include talking to your health-care provider concerning specific blood, breath, and/or digestive bacteria tests that can be performed to check for conditions that may be causing the acid reflux.

If challenged with reflux, you may want to refrain from eating or drinking products containing refined white sugar, fried foods, dairy fat, red and processed meat, citrus fruit, tomato and tomato products, pineapple, hot chili peppers, chocolate, onions, and garlic. Also avoid the consumption of products containing gluten (wheat, barley, rye, and triticale); gluten has been known to aggravate reflux. Eat only certified gluten free oats and other gluten free foods for a specified period of time and measure the results. An increase in water intake and foods with high water content such as cucumbers have very soothing effects on acid reflux, helping to balance stomach pH. Reducing stress is critically important in properly managing acid reflux. Talk to your health-care provider concerning these decisions.

Stomach: I am a part of the abdomen—not the entire abdomen as so many individuals mistakenly think. I'm located on the left side of the upper abdomen. Food enters into me via the esophagus, and I secrete the appropriate acids and enzymes to digest the food I receive. I rumble, gurgle, and contract to move food from me to the small intestine, where the inner walls of the small intestines absorb the vast majority of the nutrients and then pass them into the bloodstream. Some of the health conditions that affect me are gastric ulcer (lining deterioration), stomach cancer, gastritis (inflammation), and other health conditions. Upper endoscopy and pH testing are two exams used to review my health condition.

Foods rich in beta-carotene, such as carrots and sweet potatoes, are excellent aids for maintaining stomach health. Fresh fruits and vegetables, except those that may cause GERD issues, are highly recommended; the sulphur content in cabbage reduces the risk and severity of ulcers in support of stomach health. For my good health, avoid processed meat products, such as hot dogs, sausages, bacon, and ham; also avoid salty food and excessive salt consumption.

Colon: I'm an important part of the digestive tract, which includes the esophagus, stomach, small and large intestines, rectum, and anus. I'm also known as the large intestine and play a major role in eliminating waste from the body. I absorb the water, salt, and some of the nutrients from the foods you eat and move the remaining matter into the rectum for elimination through the final portal of the digestive tract, the anus. If waste is not properly eliminated, it can create poisonous and inflammatory disease issues in the body. The bacteria in the digestive system are known as the gut microbiota (also known as gut flora); bad bacteria are known as pathogens. Many health researchers and providers historically, as well as today, believe that the health of the body begins in the gut.

I'm home to an abundance of good bacteria that provides support for several functions including the digestion of food, absorption of nutrients and water, standing guard against the increase or growth of bad bacteria, and aiding the health of the immune system. The use of antibiotics can destroy some of my good bacteria, which can impact the bacteria's ability to properly perform these duties. According to healthyeating.sfgate.com, when the good bacteria is destroyed, the bad bacteria can increase, impairing the colon's ability to absorb nutrients and water, which can cause watery bowel movements commonly known as diarrhea. It's critically important that I regularly receive healthy fresh foods such as fruits and vegetables to strengthen and protect my good bacteria. Food sources classified as prebiotics (specific non-digestible carbohydrate fiber) can survive the travel into the colon intact and have the ability to support probiotics in its work to sustain good bacteria. These food sources include bananas, blueberries, apples, onions, garlic, artichoke, asparagus, sweet potatoes, carrots, beans, oats, and others.

It's important to limit the consumption of unhealthy saturated fat contained largely in animal food products, which is not easily eliminated from the colon region; limiting the use of tobacco and alcohol products is also important in maintaining colon health. Foods rich in antioxidant phytonutrients, such as beta-carotene and selenium, are great supports in reducing the risk of colon disease. Fresh fruits and vegetables contain important fiber to facilitate the proper function and movement of food and toxins through the digestive tract in support of colon health. Fruits such as apples, pears, blueberries, oranges, and bananas are great. Broccoli, sweet potatoes, peas, black beans, collards, spinach and other dark green leafy vegetables, brown rice, and oatmeal also protect me from colorectal disease. Folate (a B vitamin) is also important in increasing colon health. Drink plenty of fresh water to also aid the movement of foods through the digestive tract, especially when eating large amounts of fiber.

It's important to note that individuals challenged with irritable bowel syndrome (gastrointestinal discomfort, diarrhea, and constipation) should avoid common trigger foods, including cruciferous vegetables, such as broccoli, cabbage, brussels sprouts, collard greens, and kale; onions and garlic; insoluble fiber, such as wheat bran cereals, popcorn, and whole-grain products; alcohol, dairy, caffeinated, and carbonated beverages; chocolate; fatty and fried foods; and sugar-filled desserts as well as sweeteners such as fructose syrup and sorbitol. If this is a concern, talk to your health-care provider.

It's also critically important to mention that obesity, inactivity, high saturated fat consumption including red meats and processed red meats particularly grilled or cooked at high temperatures, and high levels of insulin in the blood are contributing factors to the increased risk of colon cancer. High insulin levels and conditions such as insulin resistance may promote the growth of certain tumors, including tumors in the colon according to the National Cancer Institute as reported by the Rush Medical Center in Chicago.

According to the Prevent Cancer Foundation, African Americans have the highest rate of colon cancer in the United States and are less likely to live five years or more following diagnosis, which is less than other ethnic groups; the cancer is often diagnosed in late stages. The American Cancer Society indicates scientific studies reveal that individuals diagnosed with colon cancer coupled with diabetes have an increased risk of dying. Please see your health-care provider to receive information concerning regular colon screenings.

Joints: I'm made of connective tissue and cartilage and am located in the area where two bones are joined together to accomplish movement. I join bones in the arms, legs, ankles, knees, shoulder, neck, hands, fingers, feet, toes, hips, and other places in the body. I sometimes experience pain, swelling, inflammation, and other discomfort caused by health conditions such as arthritis, gout, bursitis, cancer, dislocation, and several other bone and joint conditions. The deterioration of my cartilage between bones is a fairly common health condition that also creates pain for me. Movement and exercise are important for keeping me and my bones healthy; bicycling, walking, and swimming are great for joint movement. Weight reduction can also relieve pain and stress in joints.

Foods rich in vitamins A, C, and E, such as oranges, strawberries, blueberries, cherries, pineapple, carrots, tomatoes, broccoli, brussels sprouts, kale, collard greens, red bell peppers, avocados, and others are helpful in reducing the risk of inflammatory joint-health conditions. Foods containing rich sources of omega 3 fatty acids such as olive oil, salmon, sardines, walnuts, sunflower seeds, and pumpkin seeds are also good for me. Also eat plenty of green leafy vegetables for calcium and vitamin D, garlic for cartilage protection, and healthy whole grains such as oatmeal and brown rice. Dr. Frank Hu, Harvard University School of Public Health, recommends the aforementioned foods and also recommends limiting consumption of red meat, refined white sugar, and saturated fats to improve joint health.

Muscles: There are approximately 650 of me in the body, and I am largely made up of protein and composed of 75 percent water. I help you walk, stand, sit, talk, pump blood, and breathe, and I provide support for a variety of other functions. There are three types of muscles for the support I provide: cardiac, smooth, and skeletal. My skeletal muscles are controlled as my brain voluntarily dictates; my cardiac (heart) muscles and smooth muscles naturally operate involuntarily without me having to think about calling upon them; the cardiac muscle is constantly active and works harder than any other muscle.

I am located in just about every area of the body. Some of the common health conditions I face are inflammation and weakness caused by a variety of impairments, including toxin accumulation. Regular exercise, such as walking, swimming, and bicycling, is great for my health and longevity. I operate best when essential amino acids and complete proteins (up to daily recommended levels) are present. Some of the foods that keep me strong and motivated are free-range organic eggs and chicken breast without skin for complete protein (eat moderately); wild-caught salmon and sardines; beans and whole-grain combinations; high-pectin fiber fruits, such as apples and pears, that keep toxins moving out of the body; berries, bananas, and avocados, which help reduce sodium with their higher potassium content; cherries for their calming and soothing effect; green leafy vegetables for their oxygen contribution and tissue repair support; and, of course, lots of water to keep me properly lubricated to reduce pain and stress.

Arteries: We are blood vessels that carry oxygen-rich blood away from the heart to the body's tissues, and we also carry deoxygenated blood from the heart to the lungs for a fresh supply of oxygen when depleted blood returns to the heart from the cells and tissues. Fresh, oxygenated blood then returns to the heart from the lungs via the pulmonary veins. Veins run along the same basic path as the arteries and are passageways that flow to the heart, returning the bluish-colored, deoxygenated blood to the heart from cells and tissues; smaller arteries known as capillaries connect to the veins. We expand and contract in harmony with each heartbeat; flexible muscles within us control the flow of blood and blood pressure. Some of the common health conditions we encounter are high blood pressure when we are narrowed by poor diet or other health factors, and corrosion or hardening that can impede blood flow to the brain, causing a stroke.

Foods that produce nitric oxide, which relaxes and widens blood vessels, include beets, spinach, kale, broccoli, lettuce, watermelon, and grapes. Foods rich in potassium are great for controlling blood pressure in the arteries (see potassium under minerals section). Foods rich in magnesium aid in controlling heart rhythm and blood pressure (see magnesium under minerals section); foods rich in the B vitamins folate and B6 (pyridoxine) aid the relaxation of blood vessels, creating improved blood flow (see folate and B-6 under vitamins section). Foods rich in vitamin K support proper blood clotting and also serve to balance blood calcium levels, reducing the risk of artery calcification or hardening (see vitamin K under vitamins section).

Food for Thought

- Your body components depend on you for their proper nourishment. Don't disappoint them with health-compromising and nutrient-deficient food and drink; there's a heavy price to pay when you do.
- Some of the demands on the heart include exercise, processing of unhealthy foods, stress, strenuous work or activity, and excessive weight; potassium-rich foods, such as bananas, and a reduction of sodium intake improves heart health.

- Antioxidants and healthy whole foods such as blueberries and strawberries, dark green leafy vegetables, broccoli, carrots, sweet potatoes, omega 3 fatty fish such as salmon and sardines, walnuts, and others are great nourishment for the brain.
- Dangerous and toxic metals, including aluminum, tend to settle in the brain, contributing to neurodegenerative disorders such as Alzheimer's disease; read product labels to avoid products containing any form of toxic materials such as aluminum (see the next chapter, "More Tips and Tidbits").
- Foods that produce nitric oxide serve as natural vasodilators, which relax and widen blood vessels. These foods include beets, spinach, kale, broccoli, lettuce, watermelon, and grapes.
- Limit consumption of red meat, refined white sugar, and saturated fats to improve joint health.
- The sulphur content in cabbage reduces the risk and severity of ulcers in support of stomach health,
- An increase in water intake and foods with high water content, such as cucumbers, can have a very soothing effect on acid reflux, helping to balance stomach pH.
- Heavy use of over-the-counter drugs such as acetaminophen can contribute to premature liver failure.
- Obesity, inactivity, high saturated fat consumption, and high levels of insulin in the blood are contributing factors to the increased risk of colon cancer.
- Individuals challenged with irritable bowel syndrome (gastrointestinal discomfort, diarrhea, and constipation) should avoid trigger foods such as cruciferous vegetables, including broccoli, cabbage, brussels sprouts; onions and garlic; insoluble fiber, such as wheat bran cereals, popcorn, and whole-grain products; alcohol, dairy, caffeinated and carbonated beverages; chocolate; fatty and fried foods; and sugar-filled desserts as well as sweeteners such as fructose syrup and sorbitol.

- Diabetes can lead to heart attack and stroke and is a major contributor to nerve damage and vision impairment, including blindness. Diabetes can also lead to kidney failure. Red grapes, red bell peppers, berries, apples, cabbage and other whole foods increase kidney health.
- Avoid the use of tobacco products for the health of your lungs and your children's lungs and for overall health.
- It is critically important for women to maintain a healthy weight and eat nutritious whole foods and to avoid eating unhealthy processed foods that continually increase blood sugar and insulin levels, and to limit or avoid the consumption of high fat foods such as meat, fried foods, and high-fat dairy to support breast health.
- Men should limit or avoid the consumption of red meat, high-fat dairy, and fried foods to support prostate health; avoid excessive calcium intake. Eat tomato and tomato-based foods and talk to your health-care provider prior to taking high doses of vitamin E and selenium supplements (see omega 3 under the Fat section for other prostate health information)
- Your heart, lungs, liver, brain, colon, and other body parts should be doing cartwheels and jumping jacks after you've eaten—really!

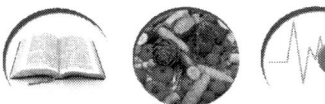

CHAPTER 15

MORE TIPS AND TIDBITS

Oxidation, inflammation, toxins, nutritional deficiency, stress, and lack of information are enemies of longevity. A few additional and repeated tips for good health include the following:

1. Eat healthy whole food such as fruits, vegetables, and whole grains with ample dietary fiber, which regulate sugar (glucose) in the blood and force toxins out of the body. Water, apples, pears, lemons, green leafy vegetables (with blood-cleansing chlorophyll), celery, carrots and carrot juice, beets, and garlic are excellent food sources for removing toxins.

2. Limit or avoid saturated and trans fat foods, such as red and processed meat and stick margarine, that contribute to colorectal disease and unhealthy fat and plaque buildup in the arteries, which contribute to heart disease and high blood pressure

3. Limit or avoid red meat, refined sugar, and saturated fats for joint health. Eat foods that reduce chronic inflammation in the joints and muscles, including pineapple, cherries, tomatoes, strawberries and blueberries, olive oil, green leafy vegetables, walnuts, wild-caught salmon and sardines, garlic, and others.

4. Eat foods rich in antioxidants, which significantly reduce cell oxidation and damage, cancer-causing free-radical development, and heart disease. Foods rich in antioxidants include blueberries, raspberries, strawberries, dark grapes, cherries,

cranberries, apples, pomegranate, broccoli, kale, beets, red bell peppers, sweet potatoes, oranges, pecans, and other foods with a significant oxygen radical absorbance capacity (ORAC) rating.

5. Stay properly hydrated with plenty of fresh water to support proper organ function and tissue moisture.

6. Experience clean, fresh outdoor air and sun each day to maintain an oxygenated environment that reduces the risk and growth of cancer cells.

7. Good health and well-being are practically impossible in an overly acidic body. While some foods have nutritional value, they should be limited due to their ability to produce and increase the body's acid level. Supply yourself with foods such as cucumbers, lemons, bananas, sweet potatoes, collard greens, kale, avocado, blueberries, apples, and carrots to maintain the proper pH (alkalinity) balance; and, of course, drink plenty of water. Limit or avoid carbonated beverages, alcohol, coffee, refined sugar, meat, corn, roasted nuts, and other acidic foods. A wide array of information is available online concerning acidic and alkaline foods; talk to your health-care provider.

8. Chew your food well! Breaking down food to its smallest components helps the stomach to better digest the food and the small intestines to better absorb its vital nutrients. The body works overtime attempting to digest food that is not well chewed. Avoid becoming overly hungry; you'll likely eat too fast, eat too much, and send improperly chewed food into the digestive system. It's OK to join the healthy nibbler society.

9. Calories are defined as "units of heat" and refer to the measured energy contained in the food you eat; the goal is to consume the appropriate number of calories in nutritious food to

support your daily function and activity. The body burns different percentages of fat and carbohydrates for fuel, depending upon your level of activity at any time. The body burns more fat calories during less intense activity, such as walking, and more carbohydrate calories when involved in more intense activity, such as jogging or running; the carb and fat fuel percentages adjust if intense activity exceeds twenty minutes or more. When involved in less intense activity, more time is needed to burn a significant number of calories.

However, for weight loss, burning fat or carbohydrate calories is not the central issue; it's simply burning more calories than you consume. According to *Back to Eden* author Jethro Kloss, the body burns approximately 1,200–1,800 calories daily even if simply relaxing or sleeping; all of your body's systems and mechanisms require energy (calories) 24-7. It's interesting to note that the body burns more calories when simply standing versus sitting. Just think of the calories you can burn in reaching your health and weight-loss goals if you simply leave the couch and become more active.

10. Watch your aluminum intake; it's very dangerous and toxic and well known to settle in the brain, contributing to neurodegenerative disorders such as Alzheimer's disease. It's often hidden in items such as pickles, cheese, baking powder, anticaking salt, nondairy creamers, deodorant, antacid tablets, buffered aspirin, and other products. Locate healthier brands that do not contain aluminum. If "alum" is anywhere in the ingredient panel, it's aluminum! You may also want to switch from aluminum cookware to stainless steel or glass cookware. Aluminum cookware loses its integrity and can break down during high-heat cooking, allowing aluminum to penetrate food; exercise caution in drinking from aluminum cans and heating foods in

aluminum foil and pie pans. It's important to note that our good friend, organic carrot juice, can aid in removing some of the toxic aluminum menace from the body.

According to the Consumer Health Organization of Canada at www.consumerhealth.org, other metals that contribute to neurological diseases are mercury, lead, cadmium, iron, and manganese. According to Natural News' online site at www.naturalnews.com, pectin-rich foods, such as green apples, bananas, beets, grapes, carrots, and citrus fruit, are great for removing toxic metals and contaminants from the body; cilantro, parsley, onions, and garlic are excellent for removing various toxic metals from the body as well. Consult with your health-care professional concerning the safe removal of metals from the body.

11. Limit or avoid the use of the microwave as much as possible. Nutrients in food are degraded and rearranged into what many in the science community classify as practically useless for the body! If using the microwave, be very careful heating food in plastic containers. The heat of the microwave releases dioxins (nasty stuff) contained in the plastic into the food; it's better to use a glass or ceramic container. Cover food in the microwave with a paper towel instead of plastic wrap; you may want to step away from the microwave oven when it's operating. It's important to mention that the Soviet Union originally banned the use of microwave ovens for well over a decade beginning in the 1970s; research and talk to your health-care provider as necessary.

12. Naturally aged flour is better for baking and retains more nutritional value for you. Flour turns a consistent white color through oxidization when allowed to age naturally. However, bleached flour is turned white with chlorine gas or peroxides (something not mentioned on the package); important nutrients are lost

during the bleaching process. Bromating flour involves adding potassium bromate to improve elasticity, giving the unaged flour better baking quality. Bleaching and bromating flour is cheaper for manufacturers. Several countries outside of the United States have banned the use of peroxides and potassium bromate—amazing! Ask your grocer about unbleached and unbromated flour brands. See more at: Earth Fare's website at www.earthfare.com.

13. If a product is labeled "low-fat," be sure to review the sugar, sodium, and food additive contents. Manufacturers often hike these contents in low-fat products to maintain the flavor when the fat is removed. Low-fat or nonfat dairy is a better choice for lowering calorie intake and reducing saturated fat in the diet; however, read the label for healthier and fewer ingredients. Talk to your health-care provider as necessary in making decisions concerning which product to consume based on your health status.

14. Heart attacks can occur when proper blood and oxygen flow is interrupted to the heart, and strokes can occur when blood and oxygen flow is interrupted to the brain. Get moving, avoid the use of tobacco, limit saturated fats, and restrict excess sodium and sugar. Be sure to include plenty of water on a daily basis and fresh, whole foods with healthy fiber, vitamins, minerals, and phytonutrients for a healthy heart and blood flow (see heart under If Body Parts Could Talk section).

15. Coffee is as popular today as it has ever been. It's amazing to watch the drive-through lines at the local coffee dispensary; you can get your favorite latte brew topped with whipped cream while on the run. It's important to know that the caffeine in coffee stimulates the central nervous system, creating short-term alertness, but it can create caffeine withdrawal characterized by

headaches and anxiety when you attempt to cease consumption. According to www.livestrong.com, caffeine also increases blood flow to the kidneys, which ultimately increases urine production and release, thereby contributing to dehydration; it's important to increase water intake when drinking coffee. The caffeine in coffee also speeds digestion, causing food to move rapidly through the intestinal tract, which may hinder the absorption of some nutrients.

16. Alcohol consumption can be very toxic to the liver and can often create an inflammatory condition known as cirrhosis, or hardening of the liver, if regularly consumed in excess. Heavy alcohol consumption is linked to a variety of health issues associated with the blood vessels, heart, brain, kidneys, breasts, stomach, pancreas, nervous system, immune system, and overall physical and psychological health. Excessive use is also known to contribute to mouth and throat cancers. According to the Centers for Disease Control and Prevention, excessive drinking between 2006 and 2010 was responsible for one in ten deaths among working-aged adults twenty to sixty-four years of age. The consumption of alcohol is a personal choice; know the facts involving its excessive and long-term use.

17. To protect yourself from chronic diseases, particularly if you're African American, you should eat well and get regular health screenings and vital information from your health-care provider; establish a relationship with a health-care provider immediately if you currently do not have one.

18. It's extremely important to increase bone mass while young because doing so slows bone loss in later years. You can assist in building bone mass by avoiding smoking, alcohol, and excessive caffeine, all of which contribute to osteoporosis, according to Jethro Kloss's *Back to Eden*.

19. Guidelines for optimal health and nutrition is accomplished by optimizing the nutrition entering your body and reducing the toxins in your body, according to *The Maker's Diet*, by Jordan S. Rubin.

As stated earlier in the book, it's important to understand the nutritional issues associated with combining various foods, commonly known as food combining. To learn more, consider visiting the Institute for Optimum Nutrition at www.ion.ac.uk/information/onarchives/foodcombiningfacts or the Acid-Alkaline Association Diet at www.acidalkalinediet.net/correct-food-combining-principles.php. Also talk to your health-care provider to learn more about food combinations and their impact on your health.

If you're interested in knowing more about foods the Bible designates as clean and unclean for consumption, Leviticus 11 and Deuteronomy 14 provide descriptions. A wide array of articles and information online is devoted to this matter, including the United Church of God's website at www.ucg.org. You can type "clean and unclean food" in the search box on the ucg.org website. Also see the article "12 Reasons Shellfish Is Unhealthy" at http://www.theluxuryspot.com/reasons-shellfish-is-unhealthy/. Choosing to refrain from eating any food type is a personal decision; talk to your health-care provider as necessary.

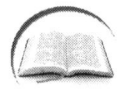 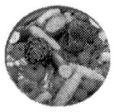 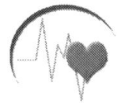

CHAPTER 16

SUMMARY

Well, you've crossed the finish line! I hope you've been inspired in a way that urges you to share with others what you've discovered as you continue your journey.

Sharing is what this book is all about. There have been many missed nights of sleep and months locked away in a small second-floor office so that this information could be assembled and shared with you. It's no secret, and as stated earlier, this work is produced through the inspiration of our Father Jehovah, our Lord and Savior Jesus, and the urging of the Holy Spirit. An interesting scripture and personal favorite speaks of sharing this way: *"When you reap the harvest of your land, do not reap to the very edges of your field or gather the gleanings of your harvest. Do not go over your vineyard a second time or pick up the grapes that have fallen. Leave them for the poor..."* (Leviticus 19:9–10 NIV).

The compelling need to share this important information concerning food and nutrition also grew from individuals encountered in various settings who repeatedly mentioned a need for nutrition information presented in a very simple and understandable way—something they could get their arms around. They needed something that spoke to them in a way that allowed them to begin to examine the benefits and risks of specific foods in relationship to their personal health interests and concerns—something they could also have in as few pages as possible that covered a wide swath of information that they could reference as needed.

Personal Message

As I mentioned in the opening pages of this book, of all the things God created in the beginning, he carefully provided food for our nourishment. Food is given to us by God. It's essential to life, but we do not worship food; we don't live to eat. We eat for health and nutrition, to strengthen ourselves to carry out the assignments and work entrusted to each of us. It is our duty and responsibility to eat sensibly and to care for the body temple that God has provided for each of us. It is written that many perish from a lack of knowledge. God doesn't want that for us; he wants us to have access to the information required for our health and well-being as we continue his assigned work. God gave us complete food and left nothing out; there is no need to attempt to improve his marvelous work.

That's where highly nutritious and whole food comes in, and that's where a lot of processed and unhealthy food choices have to take a backseat; foods that strengthen and heal have to drive the car. That's not to say we'll never eat a slice of red velvet cake with that rich cream cheese frosting or other less healthy choices seeking to hitchhike a ride; however, those are the holiday exceptions or infrequent treats and not the everyday nourishment that our heart, liver, lungs, and kidneys require and appreciate—don't get it twisted. It's critically important that people, including African American families, begin to break old habits and shift their pattern of thinking concerning food from taste to nutrition; eating for nutrition is first and essential!

You are accountable for the maintenance and well-being of your temple; dying prematurely from various chronic health conditions is often preventable. In 2010, the Center for Disease Control reported that the top four causes, comprising 57 percent, of African American deaths were attributed to chronic disease: heart disease (24.1 percent), cancer (23 percent), stroke (5.6 percent), and diabetes (4.2 percent). Cancer and heart disease were the two leading causes of death for white and Hispanic Americans as well. Below are a few enlightening, yet alarming, statistics concerning the impact of chronic disease on African Americans:

- Heart disease and stroke are the leading causes of death of women in the United States and kill nearly fifty thousand African American women annually; nearly 44 percent of African American men and 48 percent of African American women have some form of cardiovascular disease.
- Asthma affected 2.8 million African Americans in 2012 and sends African American children to the hospital at three times the rate of white children.
- African Americans have the highest rate of colon cancer in the United States and are less likely to live five years or more following diagnosis, which is less than other ethnic groups.
- Breast cancer is the leading cancer death among black women ages forty-five to sixty-four, and deaths of African American women in that age bracket were 60 percent higher than white women.
- African American men are far more likely to contract prostate disease and are twice as likely as white men to die from the disease.
- African Americans are also 80 percent more likely to be diagnosed with diabetes than whites and are twice as likely as whites to die from complications of diabetes.

The data is clear; there has to be a significant effort to trend the identified health risk downward. A diet rich in the health-sustaining natural vitamins, minerals, and phytonutrients found in fresh fruits, vegetables, healthy whole grains, beans, nuts, and seeds combined with healthier choices, such as olive oil; wild-caught fish such as salmon, mackerel, and sardines; and other nutritious foods goes a long way in establishing a barrier against debilitating chronic disease. Limiting processed foods and saturated fats, eliminating trans fats, restricting foods with high levels of added salt and sugar, greatly reducing the consumption of fried foods, avoiding tobacco, limiting alcohol and caffeine consumption, enjoying fresh water and air, reducing stress, and getting proper exercise and rest round out some of the most important physical aspects of sustaining good health. *It's worth repeating: eat well, but also get regular health screenings and secure vital information from your health-care provider; establish a relationship immediately with a health-care provider if you currently do not have one!*

A final passage of scripture connects us to the barrier that has to be established to protect you and your family from the ravaging effects of chronic disease and illness that have forcefully come into specific communities. In Exodus 12:12–13 the Lord says, *"I am the Lord. The blood will be a sign for you on the houses where you are, and when I see the blood, I will pass over you. No destructive plague will touch you."* Health is easily connected to this passage. When we eat nourishing and healing food, the plague of chronic diseases such as heart disease, cancer, stroke, diabetes, asthma, arthritis, and hypertension oftentimes have to "pass over." The blood and stain on the post of our temple is represented by the rich phytonutrients, vitamins, and minerals that provide protection to our bodies found in the wonderful, refreshing, nourishing, and healing whole foods given to us by God! Praise be to God, our Father, for inspiring us to know better so that we can certainly do better!

In Closing

Finally, I'd like to leave you with a brief story. There was a skinny little kid who grew up in a poor working family, not always having some of the things others had, sometimes not even having something under the Christmas tree. But this kid was determined to have a meaningful life in spite of his meager beginning. Things were not easily obtained in the social environment the kid grew up in, but still the young man felt there was something God would use him for one day. God can use each of us if we're open to his call and obedient to his request, even when it appears to be more than you can handle. The skinny little kid became a man and one day received his call. God's abundant blessing for good health to you and yours!

God is good all the time, and all the time God is good!

ADDITIONAL RESOURCES

Fruits and Vegetables

The World's Healthiest Foods, sponsored by the George Mateljan Foundation: http:// www.whfoods.com/foodstoc.php

"The Major Rule for Eating Fruit": http://www.mindbodygreen.com/0-4970/The-Major-Rule-for-Eating-Fruit.html

USDA National Nutrient Database for Standard Reference/Fruits and Vegetables: http://ndb.nal.usda.gov/

Dr. Decuypere's Nutrient Charts/Fruit: http://www.health-alternatives.com/fruit-nutrition-chart.html

Fruit Nutrition Facts: http://www.nutrition-and-you.com/fruit-nutrition.html,

The Health Benefits of Pears: http://www.aperfectpear.com/health-benefits-of-pears.html

Health Benefits of Limes: https://www.organicfacts.net/health-benefits/fruit/health-benefits-of-lime.html

Which Is Better for Your Health: Lemon or Lime?: http://www.livestrong.com/article/493340-which-is-better-for-the-health-lemon-or-lime/

Benefits of Fruit: https://www.organicfacts.net/health-benefits/fruit/fruits.html

The Health Risks of Sulfur Dioxide in Dried Fruit: http://healthyeating.sfgate.com/health-risks-sulfur-dioxide-dried-fruits-3921.html

The Disadvantages of Dried Fruit: http://healthyeating.sfgate.com/disadvantages-dried-fruit-3227.html

Dr. Decuypere's Nutrient Charts/Vegetables: http://www.health-alternatives.com/vegetables-nutrition-chart.html

ChooseMyPlate.gov, sponsored by the USDA: http://www.choosemyplate.gov/food-groups/vegetables_amount_table.html

Best of Sodium: http://www.fruitsandveggiesmorematters.org/sodium-in-fruits-and-vegetables

The Use of a Commercial Vegetable Juice as a Practical Means to Increase Vegetable Intake: http://www.ncbi.nlm.nih.gov/pubmed/20849620

Vegetable Nutrition Facts: http://www.nutrition-and-you.com/vegetable-nutrition.html

Benefits of Vegetables: https://www.organicfacts.net/health-benefits/vegetable/vegetables.html

Starchy Vegetables: http://www.md-health.com/Starchy-Vegetables.html

Allicin and Garlic: http://www.thirdplanetfood.com/phyt8.htm

Garlic: https://experiencelife.com/article/garlic/

Health Benefits of Chlorophyll: www.organicfacts.net/health-benefits/other/health-benefits-of-chlorophyll.html

Three Reasons Not to Eat Kale – Why for Some People It's Not the Super Food We Thought: http://www.high50.com/health/three-reasons-not-to-eat-kale

To Cook or Not to Cook Your Vegetables: http://www.everydayhealth.com/diet-and-nutrition/to-cook-or-not-to-cook-your-vegetables.aspx

Nuts, Seeds, Beans, and Grains

USDA National Nutrient Database for Standard Reference: http://ndb.nal.usda.gov/

All About Beans, North Dakota State University Extension Service: https://www.ag.ndsu.edu/pubs/yf/foods/fn1643.pdf

Health Benefits of Beans: http://www.usdrybeans.com/nutrition/health-benefits-of-beans/

Nutritional Value of Dry Beans: http://beaninstitute.com/health-benefits/nutritional-value-of-dry-beans/

The Nutritional Food Value of Beans: http://www.fitday.com/fitness-articles/nutrition/healthy-eating/the-nutritional-food-value-of-beans.html

Dr. Decuypere's Nutrient Charts/Beans: www.health-alternatives.com/legumes-nutrition-chart.html

The Hidden Dangers in Your Whole Grains, Beans, Nuts and Seeds: www.healthbeyondhype.com/the-hidden-dangers-in-your-whole-grains-beans-nuts-and-seeds-ezp-138.html

Instructions for Soaking Grains, Nuts, seeds and Legumes: www.healthbeyondhype.com/instructions-for-soaking-grains-nuts-seeds-legumes-ezp-87.html

Gluten Free Whole Grains: http://wholegrainscouncil.org/whole-grains-101/gluten-free-whole-grains

Health Benefits of Buckwheat: https://www.organicfacts.net/health-benefits/seed-and-nut/health-benefits-of-buckwheat.html

Buckwheat – December Grain of the Month: http://wholegrainscouncil.org/whole-grains-101/buckwheat-december-grain-of-the-month

11 Proven Health Benefits of Quinoa: http://authoritynutrition.com/11-proven-benefits-of-quinoa/

Is Quinoa a Complete Protein Food: http://www.livestrong.com/article/378479-is-quinoa-a-complete-protein-food/

Health Benefits of Amaranth: https://www.organicfacts.net/health-benefits/vegetable/amaranth.html

Amaranth – May Grain of the Month: http://wholegrainscouncil.org/whole-grains-101/amaranth-may-grain-of-the-month-0

Newest Research on Why You Should Avoid Soy: https://www.mercola.com/article/soy/avoid_soy.htm

Soy: The Hidden Truth About This Health Food: http://www.drmercola.com/health-tips/soy-the-hidden-truth-about-this-health-food/

Is Soy Healthy: http://wellnessmama.com/3684/is-soy-healthy/

Dr. Decuypere's Nutrient Charts/Nuts and Seeds: www.health-alternatives.com/nut-seed-nutrition-chart.html

Another Reason You Shouldn't Go Nuts on Nuts: http://chriskresser.com/another-reason-you-shouldnt-go-nuts-on-nuts/

Secrets the Nut Industry Doesn't Want You to Know: www.doctoroz.com/print/37185

Health Benefits of Nuts: Raw vs. Roasted: www.healthyeating.sfgate.com/health-benefits-nuts-raw-vs-roasted-3920.html

The World's Healthiest Foods, sponsored by the George Mateljan Foundation/Peanuts: http://www.whfoods.com/genpage.php/genpage.php?tname=foodspice&dbid=101

Nine Health Benefits of Pumpkin Seeds: http://articles.mercola.com/sites/articles/archive/2013/09/30/pumpkin-seed-benefits.aspx

Say Goodbye to Parasites: http://www.naturalhealth365.com/natural_healing/parasites.html

Living With Phytic Acid – Preparing Grains, Nuts, Seeds and Beans for Maximum Nutrition: http://www.westonaprice.org/health-topics/living-with-phytic-acid/

Why No Grains & Legumes (And Nuts?): Phytic Acid: www.paleoplan.com/2011/04-27/phytates/

Is "Frankenwheat" Fueling the Type 2 Diabetes Epidemic?: http://www.foodtrients.com/inside/is-frankenwheat-fueling-the-type-2-diabetes-epidemic/

Three Hidden Ways Wheat Makes You Fat: http://drhyman.com/blog/2012/02/13/three-hidden-ways-wheat-makes-you-fat/

Should You Worry About Wheat?: http://www.berkeleywellness.com/healthy-eating/nutrition/article/should-you-worry-about-wheat

Poultry, Fish, and Meat

The World's Healthiest Foods, sponsored by the George Mateljan Foundation/Turkey: http://www.whfoods.com/genpage.php/genpage.php?tname=foodspice&dbid=125

The World's Healthiest Foods, sponsored by the George Mateljan Foundation/Chicken: http://www.whfoods.com/genpage.php/genpage.php?tname=foodspice&dbid=116

The How and Why of Free Range Chickens: http://www.homestead.org/ReginaAnneler/Chickens/FreeRangeChickens.htm

Chicken & Turkey Nutrition Facts: http://www.fsis.usda.gov/shared/PDF/Chicken_Turkey_Nutrition_Facts.pdf

The Nutrition of Poultry: http://www.fitday.com/fitness-articles/nutrition/healthy-eating/the-nutrition-of-poultry.html

The Dangers of Farmed Fish: http://draxe.com/the-dangers-of-farmed-fish/

12 Reasons Shellfish is Unhealthy: http://www.theluxuryspot.com/reasons-shellfish-is-unhealthy/

Eating Tilapia Is Worse Than Eating Bacon: http://draxe.com/eating-tilapia-is-worse-than-eating-bacon/

Harvest of Fears: Farm Raised Fish May Not Be Free of Mercury and Other Pollutants: http://www.scientificamerican.com/article/farm-raised-fish-not-free-mercury-pcb-dioxin/

Which Fish to Pick – Farmed or Wild?: http://www.mayoclinic.org/healthy-lifestyle/nutrition-and-healthy-eating/expert-blog/farmed-vs-wild-fish/bgp-20146479

Fish and Heart Health: http://www.mayoclinic.org/healthy-lifestyle/nutrition-and-healthy-eating/expert-blog/heart-healthy-fish/bgp-20056150

Fish: Friend or Foe?: https://www.hsph.harvard.edu/nutritionsource/fish/

Health Benefits of Fish: http://www.doh.wa.gov/CommunityandEnvironment/Food/Fish/HealthBenefits

How Much Protein Is in Grilled Salmon? http://www.livestrong.com/article/361453-how-much-protein-is-in-grilled-salmon/

Red and Processed Meat Products: No Safe Amount: http://www.pcrm.org/sites/default/files/pdfs/dropthedog/Red%20and%20processed%20meat%20fact%20sheet.pdf

Every Serving of Red Meat Ups Your Breast Cancer Risk 13%: http://www.prevention.com/health/health-concerns/new-study-red-meat-ups-your-breast-cancer-risk
Risk in Red Meat? http://www.nih.gov/researchmatters/march2012/03262012meat.htm

Herbs and Spices
Herbs and Spices – Healthy Choices: http://www.veghealthguide.com/herbs-spices/
Spice of Life: Health Benefits of Spices and Herbs: http://www.fitnessmagazine.com/recipes/healthy-eating/nutrition/health-benefits-of-spices-herbs/
Cooking with Herbs and Spices "Variety Is the Spice of Life": http://www.med.umich.edu/pfans/docs/tip-2013/cookingwithherbsandspices-0513.pdf
Garden Herbs Cinnamon, Nutmeg, Ginger and Cloves: http://www.gardenherbs.org/simples/cinnamon_nutmeg_ginger_cloves.htm
Nutmeg and Cinnamon Toxicity: http://www.petpoisonhelpline.com/pet-safety-tips/nutmeg-cinnamon-toxicity/
The Health Benefits of Cinnamon, Nutmeg and Other Favorite Holiday Spices: http://articles.mercola.com/sites/articles/archive/2003/12/13/holiday-spices.aspx

Water
Functions of Water in the Body: http://www.mayoclinic.org/healthy-lifestyle/nutrition-and-healthy-eating/multimedia/functions-of-water-in-the-body/img-20005799
6 Reasons to Drink Water: http://www.webmd.com/diet/6-reasons-to-drink-water?page=1

The Benefits of Drinking Water Just After Waking Up: http://www.livestrong.com/article/446197-the-benefits-of-drinking-water-just-after-waking-up/
The Health Benefits of Water: http://www.everydayhealth.com/water-health/water-body-health.aspx
Be Unconventional – Stop Drinking with Your Meals: http://foodbabe.com/2012/02/19/be-unconventional-stop-drinking-with-your-meals/
How Fast is Water Digested?: http://www.livestrong.com/article/493343-how-fast-is-water-digested/

Oils, Butter, and Margarine
Smoke Point of Oils for Healthy Cooking: http://jonbarron.org/diet-and-nutrition/healthiest-cooking-oil-chart-smoke-points
Anti-Inflammatory Diet: How to Choose the Right Cooking Oil: http://theconsciouslife.com/omega-3-6-9-ratio-cooking-oils.htm
Butter vs. Margarine – Why I Trust Cows More Than Chemist: http://authoritynutrition.com/butter-vs-margarine/
What is Margarine and Why is it Bad For You?: http://therealfoodguide.com/what-is-margarine-and-why-is-it-bad-for-you/
The 20 Health Benefits of Real Butter: http://bodyecology.com/articles/benefits_of_real_butter.php
Health Benefits of Butter: https://www.organicfacts.net/health-benefits/animal-product/health-benefits-of-butter.html
Canola Oil: Good or Bad?: http://authoritynutrition.com/canola-oil-good-or-bad/
GMOs and Why You Should Never Use Canola Oil: http://vanessaruns.com/2011/02/08/gmos-and-why-you-should-never-use-canola-oil/
Healthy Cooking: Safflower Oil: www.healthline.com/health/safflower-oil-healthy-cooking-oil
Safflower Oil Supplement Review: http://www.clevelandclinicwellness.com/Features/Pages/SafflowerOil.aspx

What Kind of Fat is Safflower?: http://healthyeating.sfgate.com/kind-fat-safflower-8797.html

Sugar, Sweeteners, and Salt

Refined Sugar: The Sweetest Poison of All: http://www.globalhealingcenter.com/sugar-problem/refined-sugar-the-sweetest-poison-of-all

Fructose: This Addictive Commonly Used Food Feeds Cancer Cells, Triggers Weight Gain, and Promotes Premature Aging: http://articles.mercola.com/sites/articles/archive/2010/04/20/sugar-dangers.aspx

High Fructose Corn Syrup: Questions and Answers: http://www.fda.gov/Food/IngredientsPackagingLabeling/FoodAdditivesIngredients/ucm324856.htm

High Fructose Corn Syrup: www.en.wikipedia.org/wiki/High_fructose_corn_syrup

When Was Corn Syrup First Invented/Discovered? When Did They Start Using It on a Regular Basis Commercially?: http://askville.amazon.com/corn-syrup-invented-discovered-start-regular-basis-commercially/AnswerViewer.do?requestId=3834742

High Fructose Corn Syrup: Obesogenic Evil or Dietary Scapegoat, Part 1: http://nutridylan.com/2012/04/24/high-fructose-corn-syrup-obesogenic-evil-or-dietary-scapegoat-part-i/

About Sodium (Salt) – American Heart Association: http://www.heart.org/HEARTORG/GettingHealthy/NutritionCenter/HealthyEating/About-Sodium-Salt_UCM_463416_Article.jsp

How to Track Your Sodium – American Heart Association: http://www.heart.org/HEARTORG/GettingHealthy/NutritionCenter/HealthyEating/How-to-Track-Your-Sodium_UCM_449547_Article.jsp

Sodium in Diet: http://www.nlm.nih.gov/medlineplus/ency/article/002415.htm

Salt and Sodium: http://www.hsph.harvard.edu/nutritionsource/salt-and-sodium/

Food Additives

The 12 Worst Food Additives (and Where You'll Find Them): http://mindfulmomma.com/2015/01/the-12-worst-food-additives-and-where-youll-find-them.html

Other Names for MSG or Monosodium Glutamate: http://www.livestrong.com/article/377482-other-names-for-msg-or-monosodium-glutamate/

The Facts on Food Additives: Reading Nutrition Facts Food Labels: http://www.themindfulword.org/2012/nutrition-facts-food-labels/

Food Additives: https://www.ndhealthfacts.org/wiki/Food_Additives

The Dangers of MSG: http://foodmatters.tv/articles-1/the-dangers-of-msg

Related to Macronutrients and Micronutrients

Overview of Nutrition – Macronutrients and Micronutrients: http://www.merckmanuals.com/professional/nutritional-disorders/nutrition-general-considerations/overview-of-nutrition

The World's Healthiest Foods, sponsored by the George Mateljan Foundation/Essential Nutrients: http://www.whfoods.com/nutrientstoc.php

What Are Phytochemicals?: www.fruitsandveggiesmorematters.org/what-are-phytochemicals

Macronutrients: The Importance of Carbohydrate, Protein and Fat: Carbohydrates:http://www.netdoctor.co.uk/focus/nutrition/facts/lifestylemanagement/carbohydrates.htm

A Soluble Fiber Primer – Plus the Top Five Foods That Can Lower LDL Cholesterol: http://www.todaysdietitian.com/newarchives/120913p16.shtml

Soluble vs. Insoluble Fiber for IBS: http://www.everydayhealth.com/ibs/soluble-vs-insoluble-fiber-for-ibs.aspx

Soluble and Insoluble Fiber: What's the Difference?: www.webmd.com/diet/fiber-health-benefits-11/insoluble-soluble-fiber

An Apple a Day? Study Shows Soluble Fiber Boosts Immune System: http://www.sciencedaily.com/releases/2010/03/100302171531.htm

USDA National Nutrient Database for Standard Reference/Vitamins and Minerals: http://fnic.nal.usda.gov/food-composition/vitamins-and-minerals

Vitamins: http://www.vitalhealthzone.com/nutrition/vitamins/vitamins.html

http://www.mckinley.illinois.edu/handouts/macronutrients.htm

Vitamin and Minerals: http://www.healthchecksystems.com/vitamins.htm

Health Benefits of Vitamin B7 or Biotin: https://www.organicfacts.net/health-benefits/vitamins/health-benefits-of-vitamin-b7-or-biotin.html

Vitamin B7 (Biotin): Uses, Side Effects, Interactions, and Warnings: http://www.webmd.com/vitamins-supplements/ingredientmono-313-vitamin%20b7%20 (biotin).aspx?activeingredientid=313&activeingredientname=vitamin%20b7%20(biotin)

What is Vitamin B7 or Vitamin H? What is Biotin?: http://www.medicalnewstoday.com/articles/219718.php

Vitamin H (Biotin): http://umm.edu/health/medical/altmed/supplement/vitamin-h-biotin

Vitamin B12: https://www.nlm.nih.gov/medlineplus/ency/article/002403.htm

Minerals – Office on Women's Health: http://womenshealth.gov/fitness-nutrition/nutrition-basics/minerals.html

Vitamin C in Human Health is Still a Mystery – An Overview: http://www.nutritionj.com/content/2/1/7#B64

Minerals: http://www.vitalhealthzone.com/nutrition/minerals/minerals.html

Facts About Minerals: https://edis.ifas.ufl.edu/pdffiles/FY/FY89100.pdf

Calcium Content of Common Foods: http://www.iofbonehealth.org/osteoporosis-musculoskeletal-disorders/osteoporosis/prevention/calcium/calcium-content-common-foods

The Calcium Content in Kale and Collard Greens: http://www.livestrong.com/article/524516-the-calcium-content-in-kale-and-collard-greens/

7 Superfoods with Calcium: http://www.bhg.com/recipes/healthy/eating/superfoods-with-calcium/

Are Collard Greens a Better Source of Calcium Than Milk?: http://www.godairyfree.org/news/nutrition-headlines/are-collard-greens-a-better-source-of-calcium-than-milk

When Fat-Free Makes No Sense: http://blog.fooducate.com/2010/06/13/when-fat-free-makes-no-sense/

Boosting Calcium Intake with Low-Fat Yogurt: http://extension.psu.edu/publications/xk0011

Nutrients in Light Sour Cream: http://healthyeating.sfgate.com/nutrients-light-sour-cream-1827.html

New Recommended Daily Amounts of Calcium and Vitamin D: https://www.nlm.nih.gov/medlineplus/magazine/issues/winter11/articles/winter11pg12.html

MSM Health Benefits May Be Related to Its Sulfur Content: http://articles.mercola.com/sites/articles/archive/2013/03/03/msm-benefits.aspx

Selenium: http://www.vitalhealthzone.com/nutrition/minerals/selenium.html

Selenium and Vitamin E Supplements Can Increase Risk of Prostate Cancer In Some Men:
https://www.fredhutch.org/en/news/releases/2014/02/selenium-and-vitamin-e-supplements-can-increase-risk-of-prostate-cancer-in-some-men.html

Iodine: https://www.bda.uk.com/foodfacts/Iodine.pdf

Health Benefits of Iodine: https://www.organicfacts.net/health-benefits/minerals/health-benefits-of-iodine.html

Chloride: http://www.vitalhealthzone.com/nutrition/minerals/chloride. html

Chromium: http://umm.edu/health/medical/altmed/supplement/ chromium

Potassium: http://www.vitalhealthzone.com/nutrition/minerals/potassium. html

Electrolyte Imbalance – Too Much or Too Little Potassium: http://www. healthcommunities.com/electrolyte-imbalance/too-much-potassium-too-little-potassium_jhmwp.shtml

Health Benefits of Potassium: https://www.organicfacts.net/health-benefits/minerals/health-benefits-of-potassium.html

The Little Known (But Crucial Difference) Between Folate and Folic Acid: https://chriskresser.com/folate-vs-folic-acid/

Beta-carotene: https://www.nlm.nih.gov/medlineplus/druginfo/ natural/999.html

Beta-carotene: https://umm.edu/health/medical/altmed/supplement/ betacarotene

The World's Healthiest Foods, sponsored by the George Mateljan Foundation – Which is Better Monounsaturated Fats or Polyunsaturated Fats?: http://whfoods.org/genpage.php?tname=dailytip&dbid=304

Choosing Healthy Fats: http://www.helpguide.org/articles/healthy-eating/choosing-healthy-fats.htm

Does Excess Protein Turn to Fat? – An Anatomy Lesson: http://1stholistic. com/nutrition/hol_nutr_does-excess-protein-turn-to-fat.htm

Protein: http://www.hsph.harvard.edu/nutritionsource/what-should-you-eat/protein/

Protein – Iowa State University Extension and Outreach: www.extension. iastate.edu/humansciences/protein

Does the Body Store Protein?: www.livestrong.com/article/413631-does-the-body-store-protein/

Protein and Heart Health – American Heart Association: http://www.heart.org/HEARTORG/Conditions/More/MyHeartandStrokeNews/Protein-and-Heart-Health_UCM_434962_Article.jsp

The Protein Myth: https://www.pcrm.org/health/diets/vsk/vegetarian-starter-kit-protein

Does Eating Protein Burn Fat?: http://healthyeating.sfgate.com/eating-protein-burn-fat-7175.html

Dr. Decuypere's Nutrient Charts/Meat Protein: www.health-alternatives.com/meat-protein-nutrition-chart.html

If Body Parts Could Talk

How the Healthy Heart Works – American Heart Association: http://www.heart.org/HEARTORG/Conditions/CongenitalHeartDefects/AboutCongenitalHeartDefects/How-the-Healthy-Heart-Works_UCM_307016_Article.jsp

Human Heart: Anatomy, Function & Facts: http://www.livescience.com/34655-human-heart.html

Human Brain: Facts, Anatomy & Mapping Project: http://www.livescience.com/29365-human-brain.html

Picture of the Liver: http://www.webmd.com/digestive-disorders/picture-of-the-liver

Body Maps – Liver: http://www.healthline.com/human-body-maps/liver

9 Essential Facts About Your Liver: http://www.everydayhealth.com/news/facts-about-your-liver/

Lung Anatomy: http://www.medicinenet.com/lungs_design_and_purpose/article.htm

How the Lungs and Respiratory System Work: http://www.webmd.com/lung/how-we-breathe

Anatomy and Function of the Normal Lung: http://www.thoracic.org/copd-guidelines/for-patients/anatomy-and-function-of-the-normal-lung.php
How Lungs Work: http://www.lung.org/your-lungs/how-lungs-work/
Picture of the Kidneys: http://www.webmd.com/urinary-incontinence-oab/picture-of-the-kidneys
Definition of Kidney: http://www.medicinenet.com/script/main/art.asp?articlekey=4103
Diabetes and Kidney Disease: http://www.nlm.nih.gov/medlineplus/ency/article/000494.htm
The Kidneys and How They Work: http://www.niddk.nih.gov/health-information/health-topics/Anatomy/kidneys-how-they-work/Pages/anatomy.aspx
African Americans and Kidney Disease: https://www.kidney.org/news/newsroom/factsheets/African-Americans-and-CKD
Foods to Avoid With Bad Kidneys: http://www.livestrong.com/article/39928-foods-avoid-bad-kidneys/
Top 15 Healthy Foods for People with Kidney Disease: http://www.davita.com/kidney-disease/diet-and-nutrition/lifestyle/top-15-healthy-foods-for-people-with-kidney-disease/e/5347
Pancreas: Function, Location & Diseases: http://www.livescience.com/44662-pancreas.html
Pancreas Function: What Does the Pancreas Do?: http://www.medicalnewstoday.com/articles/10011.php
Foods That Will Heal the Pancreas: http://www.livestrong.com/article/36490-foods-heal-pancreas/
Susan G. Komen – What Everyone Should Know. Facts and Statistics: http://ww5.komen.org/BreastCancer/FactsandStatistics.html
Susan G. Komen – Let's Start With the Basics. What Is Breast Cancer?: http://ww5.komen.org/BreastCancer/WhatisBreastCancer.html
Black Women and Breast Cancer – Surviving Breast Cancer Through Early Detection and Diagnosis: http://www.bwhi.org/issues-and-resources/black-women-and-breast-cancer/

Insulin Breast Cancer Connection: Confirmatory Data Set the Stage for Better Care: http://jco.ascopubs.org/content/29/1/7.full

Fat and Hormonal Effects: https://www.pcrm.org/health/cancer-resources/diet-cancer/nutrition/fat-and-hormonal-effects

Eating Unhealthy Food: http://www.breastcancer.org/risk/factors/unhealthy_food

12 Foods for Breast Cancer Prevention: http://www.everydayhealth.com/breast-cancer-pictures/foods-for-breast-cancer-prevention.aspx#05

What Is the Prostate: http://www.webmd.com/men/what-is-the-prostate#2

What Does the Prostate Gland Do?: http://www.livescience.com/32751-what-does-the-prostate-gland-do.html

Tips for a Healthy Prostate: http://www.mensfitness.com/training/pro-tips/tips-healthy-prostate

Definition of Esophagus: http://www.medicinenet.com/script/main/art.asp?articlekey=3326

Picture of the Esophagus: http://www.webmd.com/digestive-disorders/picture-of-the-esophagus

Foods That Are Good for the Esophagus: http://www.livestrong.com/article/474477-foods-that-are-good-for-the-esophagus/

Medications Linked to GERD: http://www.everydayhealth.com/gerd/treating-gerd/medications-that-worsen-reflux.aspx

8 Foods That Cause Acid Reflux: http://www.globalhealingcenter.com/natural-health/foods-that-cause-acid-reflux/

3 Simple Steps to Eliminate Heartburn and Acid Reflux: http://drhyman.com/blog/2010/07/17/3-simple-steps-to-eliminate-heartburn-and-acid-reflux/

Picture of the Stomach: http://www.webmd.com/digestive-disorders/picture-of-the-stomach

The Stomach and Its Role in Digestion: http://www.laparoscopic.md/digestion/stomach

Body Map – Stomach: http://www.healthline.com/human-body-maps/stomach

What Does the Small Intestine Do?: http://www.news-medical.net/health/What-Does-the-Small-Intestine-Do.aspx

Small Intestine Function, Anatomy & Diagram – Body Maps: http://www.healthline.com/human-body-maps/small-intestine

What Is the Colon?: http://preventcancer.org/prevention/preventable-cancers/colorectal-cancer/what-is-the-colon/

The Case for Healthy Bowels: The Vital Connection Between Your Gut and Your Health: http://articles.mercola.com/sites/articles/archive/2009/04/18/probiotics-the-case-for-healthy-bowels.aspx

What Happens to Digestion When Good Bacteria in the Body Are Out of Balance: http://healthyeating.sfgate.com/happens-digestion-good-bacteria-body-out-balance-2678.html

Seven Foods to Supercharge Your Gut Bacteria: http://www.pcrm.org/media/online/sept2014/seven-foods-to-supercharge-your-gut-bacteria

Blueberries Can Help Counteract Intestinal Diseases: http://articles.mercola.com/sites/articles/archive/2010/03/04/blueberries-counteract-intestinal-diseases.aspx

4 Habits For a Healthy Gut: http://www.cnn.com/2014/06/18/health/good-gut-bacteria/

The Best Prebiotic Foods For Optimal Digestive Health: http://www.onegreenplanet.org/natural-health/best-prebiotic-foods-for-optimal-digestive-health/

What is the Function of the Colon?: http://www.puristat.com/coloncleansing/colonfunction.aspx

How to Maintain a Healthy Colon: www.foodmatters.tv/articles-1/how-to-maintain-a-healthy-colon

Increased Blood Glucose and Insulin, Body Size, and Incident Colorectal Cancer: http://jnci.oxfordjournals.org/content/91/13/1147.long

Eating for a Healthy Colon: https://www.rush.edu/health-wellness/discover-health/eating-healthy-colon

Diabetes and Colon Cancer: An Emerging Link: mhttp://www.cancer.org/research/acsresearchupdates/coloncancer/diabetes-and-colon-cancer-an-emerging-link

Foods to Choose If You Have Mixed Irritable Bowel Syndrome: https://my.clevelandclinic.org/health/diseases_conditions/hic_Irritable_Bowel_Syndrome _IBS/hic_Foods_to_Choose_if_You_Have_Mixed_Irritable_Bowel_Syndrome

Foods to Avoid with IBS: http://www.healthline.com/health/digestive-health/foods-to-avoid-with-ibs

7 Day Natural IBS Relief: http://medical-dictionary.thefreedictionary.com/irritable+bowel+syndrome

Definition of Joint: http://www.medicinenet.com/script/main/art.asp?articlekey=4074 Caring for Your Joints: http://www.webmd.com/arthritis/caring-your-joints

Foods That Fight Inflammation: http://www.health.harvard.edu/staying-healthy/foods-that-fight-inflammation

Muscular System: Facts, Functions & Diseases: http://www.livescience.com/26854-muscular-system-facts-functions-diseases.html

Healthy Muscles Matter: http://www.niams.nih.gov/health_info/kids/healthy_muscles.asp

Definition of Artery: http://www.medicinenet.com/script/main/art.asp?articlekey=2339 What Are Arteries? - Function & Definition: http://study.com/academy/lesson/what-are-arteries-function-definition-quiz.html

What Is the Difference Between arteries, Vessels, Blood Vessels and Capillaries?: http://www.wisegeek.org/what-is-the-difference-arteries-veins-blood-vessels-and-capillaries.htm

List of Foods High in Nitric Oxide: http://www.livestrong.com/article/465685-list-of-foods-high-in-nitric-oxide/

Data and Statistics

National Vital Statistics report – Deaths: Leading Causes for 2010: www.cdc.gov/nchs/data/nvsr/nvsr62/nvsr62_06.pdf

Americans Not Eating Enough Fruits and Vegetables: http://www.medicalnewstoday.com/articles/296677.php

Alcohol Use and Your Health: http://www.cdc.gov/alcohol/fact-sheets/alcohol-use.htm

Diabetes and African Americans: http://minorityhealth.hhs.gov/omh/browse.aspx?lvl=4&lvlID=18

African Americans Heart Disease and Stroke Fact Sheet: http://www.cdc.gov/dhdsp/data_statistics/fact_sheets/fs_aa.htm

Heart Disease in African-American Women: https://www.goredforwomen.org/about-heart-disease/facts_about_heart_disease_in_women-sub-category/african-american-women/

Colorectal Cancer – What African Americans Need to Know: http://preventcancer.org/prevention/preventable-cancers/colorectal-cancer/african-americans/

Prostate Cancer Grows Faster and More Aggressively in Black Men, SOM Research Finds: http://prognosis.med.wayne.edu/article/prostate-cancer-grows-faster-and-more-aggressively-in-black-men-som-research-finds

Asthma and African Americans: http://minorityhealth.hhs.gov/omh/browse.aspx?lvl=4&lvlid=15

Important Health Information

Understanding Free Radicals and Antioxidants: http://www.healthchecksystems.com/antioxid.htm

Selenium Supplements and Prostate Cancer: http://www.drsinatra.com/selenium-supplements-and-prostate-cancer/

Selenium, Vitamin E Supplements Increase Prostate Cancer Risk: http://www.health.harvard.edu/blog/selenium-vitamin-e-supplements-increase-decrease-prostate-cancer-risk-201402287059

Is Your Body Too Acidic?: www.bottomlinehealth.com/is-your-body-too-acidic/

Neural Tube Defects: http://www.nlm.nih.gov/medlineplus/neuraltubedefects.html

Resveratrol Summary – Linus Pauling Institute: http://lpi.oregonstate.edu/mic/dietary-factors/phytochemicals/resveratrol

Alkaline Foods – Reducing the Strain on the Body's Acid-Detoxification System: http://www.acidalkalinediet.net/alkaline-foods.php

The Healthiest Choice: Top 10 Alkaline Foods for Your Diet: http://vividlife.me/ultimate/4948/the-healthiest-choice-top-10-alkaline-foods-for-your-diet/

Cholesterol: Top Foods to Improve Your Numbers: http://www.mayoclinic.org/diseases-conditions/high-blood-cholesterol/in-depth/cholesterol/art-20045192

Why I'm Concerned About the Dangers of Aluminum: www.globalhealingcenter.com/heavy-metals/dangers-of-aluminum

Top Foods That Chelate the Body of Heavy Metals: http://www.naturalnews.com/038670_heavy_metals_chelation_foods.html

Chelation Therapy for Alzheimer's Disease: http://www.consumerhealth.org/articles/display.cfm?ID=19990303214451

The High Protein Myth and Aluminum Dangers: http://www.temcat.com/001-TC%20Letters/High%20Protein%20Myth-Aluminum%20Dangers.pdf

Alzheimer's and Parkinson's Disease – Detoxification Is Essential: http://www.chimachine4u.com/aluminum.html

The Health Dangers of Artificial Sweeteners: http://www.globalhealingcenter.com/nutrition/artificial-sweeteners

The Case for Healthy Bowels: The Vital Connection Between Your Gut and Your Health: rhttp://articles.mercola.com/sites/articles/archive/2009/04/18/probiotics-the-case-for-healthy-bowels.aspx

Why Did the Russians Ban an Appliance Found in 90% of American Homes?: http://articles.mercola.com/sites/articles/archive/2010/05/18/microwave-hazards.aspx

The Hidden Hazards of Microwave Cooking: http://www.health-science.com/microwave_hazards.html

Why Did the Soviet Union Ban the Use of Microwave Ovens?: http://russia-insider.com/en/why-did-russia-ban-use-microwave-ovens/5978

Top 15 Cleansing Foods: http://www.care2.com/greenliving/top-15-cleansing-foods.html

Potato Plan Poisoning – Green Tubers and Sprouts: https://www.nlm.nih.gov/medlineplus/ency/article/002875.htm

Alcohol's Effect on the Body: http://www.niaaa.nih.gov/alcohol-health/alcohols-effects-body

Effects of Coffee on Digestion: http://www.livestrong.com/article/487850-effects-of-coffee-on-digestion/

Busting the Great Myths of Fat Burning: http://www.dummies.com/how-to/content/busting-the-great-myths-of-fat-burning.html

How Wheat is Slowly Killing Millions of People: www.naturalhealth365.com/food_news/wheat.html

7 Gluten Grain Products That Can Fool You (and Make You Sick): http://celiacdisease.about.com/od/Gluten-Free-Grains/fl/Products-Not-Gluten-Free.htm

6 Reasons Why Gluten is Bad For Some People: http://authoritynutrition.com/6-shocking-reasons-why-gluten-is-bad/

Is it Gluten Free? A Basic Diet Guide for Celiacs: http://www.glutenfreeliving.com/gluten-free-foods/diet/basic-diet/

What is Celiac Disease? https://celiac.org/celiac-disease/what-is-celiac-disease/

Food Myths Debunked: Fried Foods are Too Fatty and Unhealthy: http://www.fitday.com/fitness-articles/nutrition/healthy-eating/food-myths-debunked-fried-foods-are-too-fatty-and-unhealthy.html

Why Frying Food Is Unhealthy: http://www.livestrong.com/article/440500-why-frying-food-is-unhealthy/

Hydrogenate Fats (Partially Hydrogenated Trans Fats): http://www.drgangemi.com/healthtopics/hydrogenatedfats/

Glycemic index: www.en.wikipedia.org/wiki/Glycemic_index

Heart Disease and Homocysteine: www.webmd.com/heart-disease/guide/homocysteine-risk

Taming Elevated Triglycerides, Insulin Resistance, and Syndrome X: www.drmcdougall.com/misc/2003nl/030100putamingelevatedtriglycerides.htm

Can Drinking Fruit Juice Elevate Triglycerides? http://healthyeating.sfgate.com/can-drinking-fruit-juice-elevate-triglycerides-10065.html

Food Combining – Facts & Fallacies: www.ion.ac.uk/information/onarchives/foodcombiningfacts

How to Avoid Added Nitrates and Nitrites In Your Food: http://www.healthychild.org/how-to-avoid-added-nitrates-and-nitrites-in-your-food/

Bragg Organic Apple Cider Vinegar FAQ: http://bragg.com/products/bragg-organic-apple-cider-vinegar-FAQ.html

Synthetic Nitrogen Fertilizers: http://www.organicvalley.coop/why-organic/synthetic-fertilizers/

Organic Farming Reliant on Synthetic Nitrogen: http://www.biofortified.org/2013/12/organic-farming-reliant-on-synthetic-nitrogen/

Important Terms:
Whole Food: https://en.wikipedia.org/wiki/Whole_food
Organic FAQ: http://www.organic.org/home/faq

Natural and Organic Foods: http://www.fda.gov/ohrms/dockets/
dockets/06p0094/06p-0094-cp00001-05-Tab-04-Food-Marketing-
Institute-vol1.pdf
Food, Genetically Modified: http://www.who.int/topics/food_
genetically_modified/en/
Genetically Engineered Foods: http://umm.edu/health/medical/ency/
articles/genetically-engineered-foods
Genetically Modified Organisms – FAQ: http://www.nongmoproject.
org/about-gmos-2/
What Is the Function of Cholesterol in the Body?: http://www.livestrong.
com/article/31887-function-cholesterol-body/
Cholesterol & Bile Salts: http://www.livestrong.com/article/287185-
cholesterol-bile-salts/
High Cholesterol: http://www.mayoclinic.org/diseases-conditions/
high-blood-cholesterol/basics/definition/con-20020865
Cholesterol: Causes, Symptoms, and Treatments for High Cholesterol:
http://www.medicalnewstoday.com/articles/9152.php
A Comprehensive Guide on Ideal Cholesterol Levels: http://www.
cholesterolmenu.com/cholesterol-levels-chart/
What Are Enzymes?: http://www.novozymes.com/en/about-us/our-
business/what-are-enzymes/Pages/default.aspx
Enzymes: http://medical-dictionary.thefreedictionary.com/Hormone
Probiotics and Prebiotics: Health Claim Substantiation: http://www.
ncbi.nlm.nih.gov/pmc/articles/PMC3747744/
Digging into Probiotics: Experts Look at Foods' Bacteria and Health Claims:
http://www.livescience.com/46298-the-lowdown-on-probiotics.
html
The Definition of Probiotics: 12 Years Later: http://www.
gutmicrobiotaforhealth.com/definition-probiotics-twelve-years-
later-6455
Fiber and Prebiotics: Mechanisms and Health Benefits: http://www.
ncbi.nlm.nih.gov/pmc/articles/PMC3705355/

Facts and Functions of Prebiotics, Probiotics, and Synbiotics – Kansas State University Research and Extension: http://www.k-state.edu/humannutrition/newsletters/nutrition-news/nutritionnews-documents/Prebiotics.pdf

Macrobiotics: A Way of Life: http://www.vanderbilt.edu/AnS/psychology/health_psychology/macrobiotics.htm

Macrobiotic Diet: http://www.webmd.com/diet/macrobiotic-diet

http://science.howstuffworks.com/dictionary/chemistry-terms/enzymes-info.htm

Metabolic Disorders: http://www.nlm.nih.gov/medlineplus/metabolicdisorders.html

Metabolism and Weight Loss: How You Burn Calories: http://www.mayoclinic.org/healthy-lifestyle/weight-loss/in-depth/metabolism/art-20046508

Metabolic Syndrome: http://www.mayoclinic.org/diseases-conditions/metabolic-syndrome/basics/definition/con-20027243

Metabolic Syndrome - Symptoms and Diet: http://www.medicinenet.com/metabolic_syndrome/article.htm

Electrolytes: http://www.nlm.nih.gov/medlineplus/ency/article/002350.htm

What Are Electrolytes: http://www.medicalnewstoday.com/articles/153188.php

How to Balance your pH to Heal Your Body: www.mindbodygreen.com/0-6243/How-toBalance-Your-pH-toHeal-Your-Body.html

pH: https://en.wikipedia.org/wiki/PH

Your Three Natural Body Cycles: This is Known As the Circadian Rhythms: www.blissreturned.wordpress.com/2012/01/17/your-three-natural-body-cycles-this-is-known-as-the-circadian-rhythms

Nutrition Influences Metabolism Through Circadian Rhythms – University of California, Irvine: http://news.uci.edu/press-releases/nutrition-influences-metabolism-through-circadian-rhythms-uci-study-finds/

Other Important and Inspiring Literature

Boutenko, Victoria. *Green for Life*. Raw Family Publishing. Ashland, Oregon, 2005.

Crocker, Pat, and Susan Eagles. *The Juicing Bible*. Robert Rose, Inc., Toronto, Canada, 2000.

Gregory, Dick. *Dick Gregory's Natural Diet for Folks Who Eat: Cookin' with Mother Nature*. Perennial Library, Harper & Row Publisher, New York, NY, 1973.

Kirschmann, John D. Nutrition Almanac, Better Life Through Better Nutrition, McGraw-Hill Paperback Edition, New York, NY, 1973.

Kloss, Jethro. *Back, to Eden*. Revised and expanded second edition, Kloss Family Heirloom Edition. Back to Eden Books Publishing Co., Loma Linda, California, 1992.

Melcombe, Lynne. *Health Hazards of White Sugar,* Alive Books, Vancouver, Canada, 2000.

Rubin, Jordan S. *The Maker's Diet: The 40-Day Health Experience That Will Change Your Life Forever*. The Berkley Publishing Group, New York, NY, 2005.

Waldrop, John, and Janice McCall Failes. *Natural Health and Wellness Encyclopedia*. FC&A Publishing, Peachtree City, Georgia, 1988.

Winter, Ruth. *A Consumer's Dictionary of Food Additives*. Completely revised and updated sixth edition. Three Rivers Press, New York, NY, 2004.

Wright, Henry W. *A More Excellent Way: Be In Health*, *Spiritual Roots of Disease/Pathways to Wholeness.* Pleasant Valley Publications, Thomaston, Georgia, 2003.

Wright, Keith T. *The Sweet Fetish: Sugar and Its Affect on You, Your Emotions and Your Health.* Published by Keith T. Wright, Philadelphia, Pennsylvania, 1991.

INDEX

A

D

E

F

G

H